T0271430

ROUTLEDGE LIBRARY EDITIONS: THE ADOLESCENT

Volume 8

SOCIAL WORK WITH ADOLESCENTS

SOCIAL WORK WITH ADOLESCENTS

Edited by
RAY JONES
and
COLIN PRITCHARD

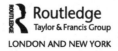

Routledge
Taylor & Francis Group

LONDON AND NEW YORK

First published in 1980 by Routledge & Kegan Paul Ltd

This edition first published in 2023
by Routledge
4 Park Square, Milton Park, Abingdon, Oxon OX14 4RN

and by Routledge
605 Third Avenue, New York, NY 10158

Routledge is an imprint of the Taylor & Francis Group, an informa business

ISBN: 978-1-032-37655-4 (Set)
ISBN: 978-1-032-37819-0 (Volume 8) (hbk)
ISBN: 978-1-032-37824-4 (Volume 8) (pbk)
ISBN: 978-1-003-34211-3 (Volume 8) (ebk)

DOI: 10.4324/9781003342113

Publisher's Note
The publisher has gone to great lengths to ensure the quality of this reprint but points out that some imperfections in the original copies may be apparent.

Disclaimer
The publisher has made every effort to trace copyright holders and would welcome correspondence from those they have been unable to trace.

Social work
with adolescents

edited by

Ray Jones

*Lecturer in Social Work
University of Bath*

Colin Pritchard

*Director of Social Work Studies
University of Bath*

Routledge & Kegan Paul
London, Boston and Henley

First published in 1980
by Routledge & Kegan Paul Ltd
39 Store Street,
London WC1E 7DD,
9 Park Street,
Boston, Mass. 02108, USA and
Broadway House,
Newtown Road,
Henley-on-Thames,
Oxon RG9 1EN
Printed in Great Britain by
Redwood Burn Ltd, Trowbridge & Esher
© Routledge & Kegan Paul Ltd 1980

British Library Cataloguing in Publication Data

Social work with adolescents. – (Library of
social work ISSN 0305–4381).
1. Social work with youth
I. Title
II. Jones, Ray   III. Pritchard, Colin
IV. Series
362.7   HV1421

ISBN 0 7100 0633 0

Contents

Contributors

RAY JONES is Lecturer in Social Work at the University of
Bath. He has worked in mental health hostels, and as a
social worker and senior social worker in a social services
department. He has undertaken research on adolescents'
perceptions of social work, on intermediate treatment, and
on neighbourhood work, and he continues to work with children in trouble. He is author of 'Fun and Therapy: consumer and social worker perceptions of intermediate treatment' (National Youth Bureau, 1979), and he is co-author
of 'Intermediate Treatment and Social Work' (Heinemann,
1979).

COLIN PRITCHARD is Senior Lecturer, and Director of
Social Work Studies, at the University of Bath. He has
worked in adult and child psychiatry, and was previously
Lecturer in Psychiatric Social Work at the University of
Leeds. He has undertaken research on school phobia, on
the relationships between social workers and teachers, and
on the CND movement. He is involved in in-service training for social work supervisors and managers, and continues to work as a counsellor. He is co-author of 'Social
Work: Reform or Revolution?' (Routledge & Kegan Paul,
1978) and of 'The Protectors - CND Twenty Years On'
(Pergamon, 1980).

JACK DUNHAM is Lecturer in Social Psychology at the
University of Bath. He has previously worked in schools,
child guidance clinics, and with the Bristol Aeroplane Company. He is involved in both social worker and teacher
training, and is currently researching the stress experienced by 'professional helpers'. He is joint author of 'The

Nylon Spinners' (Allen & Unwin, 1971), and was Chairman of the Federation of Mental Health Workers from 1973 until 1978.

FLORENCE ROSSETTI is Lecturer in Applied Social Studies at the University of Bath. She has wide experience of community development in Italy and in the Third World, has worked as a social development officer with the Community Relations Commission, and was Director of Southwark Community Development Project. She is involved in community work consultancy with several agencies, is currently researching community work in rural areas, and was a contributor to 'Political Issues and Community Work' (Routledge & Kegan Paul, 1978).

AUDREY TAYLOR is Tutor in Social Work at the University of Bath. She has worked as a social worker in hospitals, child guidance clinics, and social services departments, and continues to carry a child guidance caseload. She has previously undertaken research on child abuse, and is curretly researching consumer perceptions of maternity services.

ANDREW KERSLAKE is Tutor in Social Work at the University of Bath. He has worked as a specialist social worker with adolescents, and as an intermediate treatment officer with responsibility for an IT Centre. He is involved in groupwork consultancy and training with several social work agencies, and is co-author of 'Intermediate treatment and Social Work' (Heinemann, 1979).

JOHN BURNS is Principal of Kingswood School, Bristol, a large community home with education. He has 30 years' experience in field and residential social work, including working as a probation officer, child care officer, and as Children's Officer with Rochdale County Borough Council. In 1963 he was awarded the MBE for his work at Stamford House Remand Home. He is a past president of the Association of Community Home Schools, and a ministerial appointee to the Personal Social Services Council.

WILLIAM GREGORY is Headmaster of the Special (Secure) Unit at Kingswood School, Bristol. He has extensive experience of teaching in state schools and in approved schools. He is a contributor to 'Residential Care: A Reader in Current Practice and Theory' (Pergamon, 1980), and is a recent past president of the Association of Community Home Schools.

GRAHAM TEMPLEMAN is Headmaster of the Assessment Centre at Kingswood School, Bristol. He qualified as a teacher, has wide experience of teaching in approved schools, and was previously Deputy Headmaster of the Regional Assessment Centre at Tennal School, Birmingham.

KEN REID is Associate Professor of Social Work at Western Michigan University, USA. In 1977 he was Visiting Professor of Social Work at the University of Bath. He has experience of individual, family and group counselling, and was awarded a doctorate in 1976 for his research on the history of groupwork. He is currently researching the 'burn-out' syndrome amongst social workers.

Chapter one

Setting the scene

Ray Jones and Colin Pritchard

Until recently the popular image of the adolescent was one
of inevitable storm and stress, so that what were seen as
the 'in-between years' of adolescene were almost, by definition, seen as a time of disturbance. This simplistic,
classical view is now rightly being questioned, and, while
not denying the irritability and occasionally irrational behaviour which adolescents may show, or evoke from others,
we would start from the premise that adolescence is a normal period of development, and that adolescent behaviour is
usually rational and understandable. Professional workers,
in particular, need to be aware of the danger of over-inter-
preting actions and behaviour, which, whilst being distressing to the adolescent and a nuisance to others, are not in
themselves 'pathological'. Such a cautious and normative
stance taken towards the adolescent enables the professional adviser to be more able to differentiate between behaviour which is particularly problematic and pathological, and
behaviour which is essentially normal. This theme is developed further in the chapter by Jack Dunham and Ray Jones
on 'Understanding Adolescence', where they explore some
of the theoretical concepts of adolescence, and discuss man
many aspects of adolescent development and behaviour.
  In this book adolescence is taken to start with puberty
and to end when adult identities and roles, such as work and
marriage, have been accepted and assimilated. The dura-
tion of the process of adolescence varies between individuals, between generations, and between cultures. For
instance, the 20-year-old who has been working for four
years, and who is married with children, may be more
readily recognised and accepted as an adult than a student
of the same age who still lives in his parents' home. Hence

1

within this text we appreciate that any comments made about adolescence must of necessity be generalised. Equally important, such generalisations need to be interpreted against the back-drop of the level of development and the social situation of each individual, and to take into account the adolescents' own perceptions of their experience. Hence any intervention with an adolescent should seek to establish a personally and culturally normal baseline from which the social worker assesses that person's situation.

Young people, of course, do get into trouble with parents and more generally with society, and they are sent to, and occasionally seek the assistance of, social workers. The particular expertise of social workers is that they can consider a range of theoretical explanations, and the associated intervention methods, which might be used to assist the adolescent. It is the ability of the social worker to adopt a range of perspectives and techniques that should characterise the important social work contribution to work with adolescents. This contribution is built on the understanding that adolescence, like any other stage of life, is an interactive process. It is the combination of, and the relationships between, the individual's physiology, his emotions, his social roles, and his material environment, which characterises that individual, and it is these interacting aspects which we need to consider in our assessments and interventions.

There are, however, two dangers for social workers in their assessment of adolescents. On the one hand they may underestimate the potential seriousness of the problem - the 'he'll grow out of it' response; on the other hand they may over-react to the presenting situation, especially when faced by a strident referrent who asserts that 'something must be done'. It is difficult to strike an appropriate balance, when in the first instance the most careful negotiations may be required to gain the co-operation of all involved, while the second situation, when it is possible to assure adolescents and adults that little is wrong, may well require considerable time and tact. This book attempts to examine some of these practical problems, and to demonstrate some of the various roles and tasks undertaken by social workers in their work with young people. A range of approaches will be explored, partly to illustrate points of similarity and overlap, and partly to highlight the different emphases of the varied forms of intervention. There are, however, two crucial omissions in the text.

The first major omission is that there can only be relatively slight discussion of the approaches of other professions, because this book focuses primarily upon <u>social work</u> with adolescents. Nevertheless we attempt to offset this deficit by Jack Dunham's chapter, which recognises the important contribution of other disciplines, while acknowledging the difficulties surrounding liaison and interaction between people of possibly differing orientations.

Two of the most important professional groups concerned with adolescents are school-teachers and the medical profession, such as general practitioners and psychiatrists. In the case of teachers, despite the occasional inter-disciplinary rivalries between them and social workers, there is evidence that they welcome social work help with those youngsters who exceed their professional skills, especially if such assistance is provided within a structure that facilitates social worker accessibility, such as school-based social workers (Pritchard and Taylor, 1979). The central importance of the school system in social work with the adolescent is increasingly recognised, and Robinson(1979) usefully explores many of the areas of common interests between school-teachers and social workers.

The medical profession, especially those doctors with a psycho-social perspective, have made a significant contribution to the understanding of adolescents, and have undoubtedly influenced much of the post-war development of social work (see, for example, Kahn and Nursten, 1964). Continued growth in psychiatric interest in adolescence has included a strong behavioural and social science approach, as is illustrated by the work of Rutter (to which we refer throughout this book) which reflects an increasing degree of multi-disciplinary activity in this field. The practical implications for such developments are discussed at some length in Chapter four, where it is stressed that all who would be involved in the life of an adolescent need to enquire which, if any, of the other disciplines might be concerned, and be prepared to consider an alternative paradigm of the other professional.

The second key omission from the book is consideration of the socio-political and ethical context in which social work is practised. That social work is part of a general political process is accepted (Butrym, 1976), though argument continues as to the nature and direction of that process (Corrigan and Leonard, 1978; Halmos, 1978). Differing political perspectives have been identified in the

various forms of social work, and the ensuing practical implications about the role of the social worker in situations
of care, control, change and conflict have been discussed
by Pritchard and Taylor (1978). It is argued that all professional activity, if it is to be rational, requires an understanding of the political contexts in which it operates.
Throughout our text only the briefest mention can be made
of these issues, which impinge not only upon the social work
service, but upon every aspect of the adolescent's life. It
would be regrettable if the reader were not reminded that
we believe the importance of economic and socio-political
factors to be self-evident. This seems to be particularly
pertinent at the present time when the current government
is re-defining some of the legislation that directly affects
adolescents and the services provided for them, and when
there has recently been a demographic peak in the number
of adolescents, but also a reduction in the public expenditure which is made available to provide services for them.

THE STRUCTURE OF THE BOOK

In continuing to set the scene it might be helpful to offer an
outline of the book. One of the key aims is to present in
one text a range of different approaches. Such a presentation avoids the more usual mode of giving just one or two
'methods', with the minimal placatory nods towards other
orientations. It is hoped that by combining varying perspectives in one book we can gain a balanced discussion of
the main trends in social work with the adolescent. In
addition it is hoped that this will allow some consideration
of elements common to all types of intervention, without
obscuring those areas of real controversy.
   The book falls into two broad areas. The first section
serves as a foundation, exploring general issues of adolescent development, and a conceptualisation of social work
practice which is illustrated by examples from work with
adolescents. This section also discusses some of the
problematic areas concerned with collaboration between
different professional groups. The second section of the
book describes in some detail a range of social work intervention which can be of value when working with young
people. The last chapter of this section examines the
impact upon the social worker of some of the specific pressures associated with work with adolescents. Finally the

editors offer a postscript, which seeks to bring together
some of the prevailing themes and looks towards future
developments.

Part I

To provide a base for the subsequent practice contributions,
Jack Dunham and Ray Jones review in Chapter two some of
the major theories related to adolescent development. In
addition they offer a working model for understanding adolescents that reflects their own practice interest. In providing this general parameter it should be emphasised, however, that there will be some overlap with those contribu-
tors who will explore those developmental features of adolescence which are of particular relevance to their practice
approach. Indeed, all the intervention papers start from a
common baseline of considering adolescence from a normative stance, and it is upon this baseline that they build their
discussion of the social work response to difficulties encountered by the adolescent.
    A second theme within the first part of the book is presen-
ted by Florence Rossetti in Chapter three. She discusses
the relevance to work with young people of concepts drawn
from the unitary approach to social work. It can be argued
that adolescents can be seen as being at the centre of a network of welfare services which have a common link through
the adolescent. Such inter-linked provisions include
health, education, employment and social services. Thus
Rossetti's consideration of the unitary approach offers a
valuable theoretical and practical model by which to analyse
many of the support and stress 'systems' that may affect
adolescents. Her chapter also highlights the interactional
nature of both adolescent development and of work with
adolescents. An important adjunct to this chapter is the
discussion of 'method' in social work, and this provides a
framework for considering the various intervention styles
presented in this book. This provocative discussion offers
a stimulating challenge by which to further the debate about
the theoretical under-pinnings of the traditional triumvirate
of social work methods.
    In Chapter four a bridge between the foundation and inter-
vention papers is given by Jack Dunham who, accepting
Florence Rossetti's discussion of the adolescent in his
social situation - a situation which might include other

agencies – reviews the problems associated with inter-professional contact and liaison. Sadly some practitioners may well ask 'what contact; what liaison?', as so often one professional group uses the other as a scapegoat for its frustrations, although we would not deny the value of conflicts which exist between some of those involved with young people, especially young people in trouble. The emphasis in this chapter is upon inter-professional communication, and strategies are offered to resolve some of the problems. Nevertheless it should be recognised that intra-disciplinary communication can be equally problematic when, for example, there is need for collaboration between a social worker with a psychotherapeutic orientation and a social work colleague who has a major allegiance towards a radical political ideology.

Part II

In the second section of the book we examine in some detail three of the main types of social work intervention. In Chapter five Audrey Taylor and Colin Pritchard explore the counselling process with the adolescent and his family. They focus upon those intensities of family interaction and development which can create considerable distress for all involved. They attempt to use, in an eclectic and integrated way, a range of psychological theories associated with different counselling strategies. They seek to maintain a balance between identification with either adolescent or parents – such a response demands a sympathetic recall by the older social worker of the adolescent experience, and an imaginative exercise by the younger social worker of what middle age means in a rapidly changing psycho-social scenario. Andrew Kerslake then looks in Chapter six at the importance of the peer group, and its potential as a base for subsequent social work with adolescents. He offers a practical exploration of some of the issues in social group work undertaken by field social workers, and comments briefly upon group work with young people in other settings. In Chapter seven Ray Jones examines the impact of the neighbourhood setting upon the adolescent, and how social work might better utilise the adolescent's experience within his neighbourhood. It is suggested that the particular value of the neighbourhood perspective is that it minimises the stigmatising and labelling processes which are experienced by many clients of the welfare services, while in addition there will be benefit to the client by maintaining and strengthening those supports that may be available within the local community.

A frequent criticism of social work texts is the apparent neglect of residential services. This may be due to a number of reasons, not least because the admission of a youngster into care is often believed to be a tacit acceptance of 'failure' by social workers, rather than seeing residential care as a valuable resource for some adolescents. It is, however, recognised that reception into care, to be an appropriate service, should be a response to carefully assessed need being matched with the potential of the service being offered, and not just, as at present, a convenient disposal of 'troublesome' children (Hoghughi, 1978b; Millham et al., 1978; Thorpe et al., 1979). Some of these issues are discussed by John Burns and his colleagues in Chapter seven, where they develop the idea of residential care being a 'second chance' for young people needing care and protection. These writers offer an essentially practice-based paper from considerable experience of working together in a community home which was a former approved school.

The penultimate chapter, by Ken Reid, draws upon the interactional theme running throughout the book to look at the impact the adolescent has upon the social worker. He explores some of the common feelings and reactions which adolescents may promote and provoke in adults. He examines how the potentially sexually and aggressively provocative adolescent might revive feelings and attitudes evolved from the worker's own adolescence, and how the adolescent may be felt to be a challenge to our own maturity, competence and professional identity. Reid's focus has evolved from a predominately counselling approach, yet it will be argued that this contribution is relevant to all methods which involve face-to-face contact with adolescents as, irrespective of one's view of adolescence, contact between adults and young people has the potential to re-arouse emotions that have their roots in the adult's own social and psychological background. This, we believe, is as axiomatic as the Delphic 'know thyself'; for unless the adult is willing to consider that the situation facing the adolescent might be different from his own, then that adult is in danger of assuming a series of norms and moral imperatives which are fallaciously based upon his own experience. Such an

unquestioning response from older people in authority
implies that their arrogance is only matched by their ignorance.

This book represents the University of Bath social work
team's response to the general editor's invitation that different schools of social work 'could speak with a collective
(but not necessarily uniform) voice' (Timms, 1975). With
colleagues from a local community home we have attempted
to offer a text that does not hide the differences in the various approaches to work with young people, but rather to
offer a collection of papers that allows consideration of
both common elements and divergences. To relate the different contributions to each other the editors briefly introduce and comment on each chapter. These remarks are
given in square brackets before the beginning of the main
text. It is hoped that the text provides some assistance in
avoiding the complaint made about social workers in a skinhead magazine: 'THEM – social workers who talk about
your "problem" and their "help", when it's just their kind
of help that is your problem!'

Part I

Understanding adolescence and social work

Chapter two

Understanding adolescence

Jack Dunham and Ray Jones

/What is adolescence? How is adolescent development
understood? How do adolescents tend to behave? These
questions are explored in this chapter, which discusses
some models of adolescence. The paper seeks to offer a
number of developmental theories which serve as a foundation for the subsequent contributions. The authors of this
chapter then go on to present a stress model of adolescent
development and, based upon a review of some of the research literature, comment upon the processes of change
that occur during adolescence./

Our concern in this chapter is to present a number of differing frameworks to help us understand the process of
adolescence, and then to discuss in more detail some of
the personal and social changes which occur as a part of
this process. We discuss five models of adolescence which
we have found to be useful frameworks to aid our understanding of adolescent development, and we are particularly
concerned to help social workers cope with the everyday
demands of adolescents rather than focusing on special
cases or unusual problems. We agree with Coleman when
he states:

> Developmental psychology has a special responsibility
> to those most immediately involved with children and
> adolescents, and it is sad but true that too many psychol-
> ogists too frequently lose sight of this fact (Coleman,
> 1974, p. ix).

11

FIVE MODELS OF ADOLESCENCE

Constitutional model

Our first explanation of adolescence is based on the biological or constitutional perspective which studies the changes
which occur in physique and physical capabilities. These
studies include the different ages at which puberty comes,
the effects of early and late development, the continuing
effects of sex differences, and the relationship between
temperament and personality.

   These studies usually indicate great individual differences in biological development. The implications of this
mean that in a group of 11- to 12-year-old girls there will
be some who have reached adolescence and begun to menstruate while others show no signs of sexual maturity, such
as the growth of breasts, nor of the spurt in growth. The
early maturing girls will tend to be bigger and stronger
than most 11- to 12-year-old boys because the adolescent
growth spurt for the male comes later. The physiological
changes have been starting earlier for each generation of
females since the beginning of this century though this tendency is now beginning to level off (Reynolds, 1976). The
average age for the onset of menstruation is now just over
13 years and the range for the beginning of their periods
for 95 per cent of all girls runs from 10 to 15 years. Some
girls therefore begin to menstruate before they leave primary school and some have not started by the time they have
completed three years in secondary school.

   Boys have also shown this trend to earlier sexual maturity and an earlier start to the growth spurt. The range of
individual differences in boys' biological development is as
wide as that for girls, for example 'acceleration in penis
growth is already over for some children at the age of
thirteen-and-a-half while for others it does not begin until
fourteen-and-a-half' (Reynolds, 1976). There are important psychological implications of these physiological facts
because some boys of thirteen to fourteen years of age have
reached sexual maturity, and have the stature and almost
the strength of an adult, and some boys of the same age are
still children. These differences can lead to considerable
adjustment difficulties in schools because 'our educational
system tends to treat pupils at a given age as if they were
all the same physiologically' (Lovell, 1973), rather than
responding to the 'physical self' of each individual. We

return again to this issue of physical development later in the chapter.

Another significant self, in the total pattern of selves which can be described as identity, is temperament, and this too has a significant constitutional basis. The importance of this perspective in understanding child and adolescent behaviour has been clearly shown in a research study carried out by Thomas (1970) and his colleagues in New York. Temperament is defined as an individual's behavioural style or tempo with respect to 'characteristics such as the regularity of their various biological cycles (sleep/waking, hunger/satiety), their adaptability in response to altered circumstances, and the intensity of their emotional responses' (Rutter, 1974, p. 79). Thomas's longitudinal study of families in New York found differences in these temperamental characteristics as early as the second month of life. Some of the children have 'markedly irregular patterns of functioning (as shown, for example, by the fact that they woke and went to sleep at unpredictable times), whose emotional responses were usually of high intensity and whose predominant mood was one of misery or irritability' (Rutter, 1974, p. 79). Other children in the study had the opposite characteristics of 'positiveness in mood, regularity in bodily functions and a low or moderate intensity of reaction' (Thomas et al., 1970, p. 5). These differences were evident ten years later and Table 2.1 illustrates the importance and permanency of the effect of temperament by selecting just one characteristic from the list provided by Thomas.

TABLE 2.1 Continuity of temperament

Temperamental quality	Rating	2 months	10 years
Intensity of reaction	Intense	Rejects food vigorously when satisfied	Tears up page of homework if one mistake is made
	Mild	Whimpers instead of crying when hungry	When a mistake is made in a model aeroplane corrects it quietly

It is clear from further research information which has been given by Thomas and Chess that their longitudinal study strongly indicates the continuity into adulthood of these temperamental differences in adolescence. They stated that 'We have been impressed by the important roles that temperament continues to play at later stages of development' (Thomas and Chess, 1977, p. 25).

Identity crises

Our second explanation of the behaviour of adolescents is that they are disturbed by crises of identity, which some may attempt to resolve by withdrawing from parents, teachers and sometimes their peers. Erikson has attempted to persuade us that young people need a period which he called a 'psychosocial moratorium' during which they can attempt to complete their search for an identity.

Erikson believes that at the end of the adolescent phase, which is the crucial one in his eight-phase theory of development, a young adult should have a firm self-concept which will enable him to continue to play a number of different roles without losing his clear awareness of personal identity. In Erikson's view an integrated person can cope with adult problems of marriage and rearing a family from the basis of a settled occupational role if he has experienced, as an adolescent, a 'diffusion of roles' in his attempts at exploration. Erikson has described this essential process in his ornate language:

> The adolescent's leaning out over any number of preci-
> pices is normally an experimentation with experiences
> which are thus becoming more amenable to self-control,
> provided they can be somehow communicated to other
> adolescents in one of those strange codes established for
> just such experiences – and provided they are not pre-
> maturely responded to with fatal seriousness by over-
> eager or neurotic adults (Erikson, 1977, p. 125).

The experimentation with different roles and identities helps adolescents to prepare themselves for the choices they have to make. They have to make choices about, and adapt to, an occupational identity as they move into employment, and there are also non-occupational choices and decisions which may be demanding and require much attention and energy. These can include considerable doubts about one's ethnic identity as a member of a minority group

in a multi-racial society, and a disturbing uncertainty
about one's sexual identity when one feels unable to play
the sexual roles presented by the mass media.   It is not
surprising that many adults perceive, and indeed expect,
all adolescents to suffer from crises of identity which need
space and time to be worked out.

Social learning model

This perspective is still widely used, but a very different
approach is steadily becoming more acceptable.   The supporters of the more recent theory are very critical of what
they term the 'adolescent myth' of inevitable confusion and
difficulties.   Rutter et al. (1976), for instance, have found
that although feelings of misery and self-depreciation are
common amongst 14-year-olds, these feelings are often not
recognised by adults, and he also found that psychiatric
disturbance is hardly any more common during adolescence
than during childhood.
     One of the strongest critics of the model of adolescent
crises is Bandura, who, quoting from his own research into
the experiences of American teenagers, has concluded that
many young people are socialised without major snags from
childhood into the roles they will play as adults.   They
know what is expected of them and they identify with these
expectations as they gradually develop the appropriate
occupational, ethnic and sexual identities.   There is no
need for a moratorium because there is no 'identity crisis'
or even a special adolescent stage to be worked through.
Bandura suggests that some adolescents behave as society
expects them to behave:
     If a society labels its adolescents as 'teen-agers' and
     expects them to be rebellious, sloppy and wild in their
     behaviour, and if this picture is repeatedly reinforced by
     the mass media, such cultural expectations may very well
     force adolescents into the role of rebel (Bandura, 1970,
     p. 24).
Much of Bandura's research has been concerned with
aggressive behaviour and his interpretation is in direct
conflict with those psycho-analytic explanations which emphasise the importance of releasing pent-up energy directly
or vicariously by, for example, watching violence on tele-
vision.   Bandura and his colleagues argue very strongly
the contrary position that seeing aggressive behaviour will

stimulate the observers to imitate the aggressive models
they have been watching (see also Belson, 1978; Eysenck,
1978). He is particularly concerned that the effects of
television are not under-estimated:

> The finding that film-mediated models are as effective as
> real-life models in eliciting and transmitting aggressive
> responses indicates that televised models may serve as
> important sources of behaviour and can no longer be ig-
> nored in conceptualisations of personality development.
> Indeed, most youngsters probably have more exposure to
> televised male models than to their own fathers. With
> further advances in mass media and audio-visual technol-
> ogy, models presented pictorially, mainly through tele-
> vision, are likely to play an increasingly influential role
> in shaping personality patterns (Bandura, 1967, p. 98).

The importance of investigating the role models offered to
adolescents can also be seen when examining the results of
a recent research project on the progress of the pupils in
twelve secondary schools in inner London. Over two thousand pupils were observed in their classrooms and they also
provided questionnaire data for the research workers
(Rutter et al., 1979). The study found that (p. 157):

> Pupils are likely to be influenced – either for good or ill
> – by the models of behaviour provided by teachers both in
> the classroom and elsewhere. These will not be restric-
> ted to the ways in which teachers treat the children, but
> may also include the ways staff interact with one another,
> and how they view the school. Our observations of good
> care of the buildings, and the willingness of teachers to
> see pupils about problems at any time, provide some ex-
> amples of positive models. Negative models would be
> provided by teachers starting lessons late and ending
> them early, and by their use of unofficial physical sanc-
> tions. If teachers react with violence to provocation
> and disruptiveness this may well encourage pupils to do
> the same.

Hence the role models offered to adolescents are of great
importance, and these also include the role models which
may be offered by social workers.

Needs model

The fourth perspective which social workers might find
useful in understanding adolescent behaviour is concerned

with attempts to satisfy needs. This theory was first pro-
pounded by Maslow (1970). In Maslow's formulation there
are five levels of needs; when level one needs are satis-
fied we can pay attention to those at level two and so we
continue to the final level:

Level 1: Physiological needs
Level 2: Security
Level 3: Acceptance
Level 4: Identity
Level 5: Self-fulfilment

The physiological needs at the base of the hierarchy have
been investigated in a number of experiments. Studies of
people who have experienced severe sleep loss have shown
significant increases in their aggressive and irrational
behaviour (Wilkinson, 1966). Studies of people who have
been subjected to very low levels of stimulation have indicated considerable effects on their ability to concentrate and
make decisions (Cooper, 1969). One important conclusion
of these experiments is that the brain may not function
effectively in conditions of boredom and monotony.

Next in Maslow's hierarchy are the security needs which
if unsatisfied may dominate adolescent thinking and behaviour. According to this view if, for instance, adolescents
are preoccupied with job security because of fears of unemployment they may be unable to concern themselves with any
other part of the work situation such as, for example, a
training course. At home they may be unable to cope with
family demands.

If both the physiological and security levels are fairly
well gratified, Maslow argues it then becomes possible for
the next need level to be reached. Now an adolescent is
aware of, and can pay attention to, his need for acceptance,
love and attention which will frequently be expressed as a
need to belong to a group. Maslow has described the
strength of this craving for satisfying inter-personal relationships:

Now the person will feel keenly as never before, the absence of friends or a sweetheart or a wife or children.
He will hunger for affectionate relations with people in
general, namely for a place in his group, and he will
strive with great intensity to achieve this goal. He will
want to attain such a place more than anything else in the
world and may even forget that once he sneered at love as
unreal or unnecessary or unimportant (Maslow, 1970,
p. 75).

Social workers will probably know adolescents who have
such strong needs to be accepted in groups of their peers
that they will conform to pressures to take part in delinquent and even violent behaviour. They may also know
adolescents who feel this need intensely because they feel
isolated at home, at school, or at work.

The identity needs are the next to appear in the hierarchy.
These include self-respect and the respect of other people.
The satisfaction of these needs leads, it has been argued,
to feelings of self-confidence and personal worth.

When these four levels of physiological, security, acceptance and identity needs have been 'largely gratified' it is
Maslow's contention that people become concerned with
self-fulfilment. Their behaviour is now motivated by the
dominant aim of personal growth 'to achieve their own potentiality' (Herzberg, 1968). They seek challenges to achieve
higher levels of competence. Their behaviour is very different from those adolescents who are still attempting to
satisfy their physiological, security, acceptance and identity needs:

When we examine people who are predominantly growth-
motivated, the coming-to-rest conceptions of motivation
becomes completely useless. In such people gratification breeds increased rather than decreased motivation,
heightened rather than lessened excitement. Rather than
coming to rest, they become more active (Maslow, 1970,
p. 201).

These views of human motivation have been attacked by
critics, for example Cofer and Appley (1964), who find them
imprecise and without acceptable research support. They
are, however, still influential and one of the most recent
formulations has been put forward by Mia Kellmer Pringle
(1974). She has proposed that children have four basic
needs: love and security, new experiences, praise and
recognition, and responsibility. In her view the first of
these is the most important and she argues that anger, hate,
vandalism and violence are common reactions amongst adolescents to feelings of rejection. These aggressive reactions are also thought to be the result of the non-satisfac-
tion of the other needs because of boring conditions at
home, school or work, where adolescents may also receive
little recognition or responsibility.

Stress model

The reactions to frustrating lives which Pringle has identified are as yet taken by only a small minority of young
people. A much larger number respond by other emotional,
behavioural and psychosomatic symptoms, and our fifth perspective in attempting to understand adolescent behaviour
and problems seeks to relate these responses to the stress
situations which young people have to cope with in their
families, at school, at work, and in the community. A high
level of unemployment is an example of a major stress situation for many adolescents which may evoke the responses of
delinquency, violence, cynicism, depression and apathy.

The response to stress situations is determined by the
resources available to an adolescent. These include his
personal strengths and weaknesses, the acceptance, recognition and support he receives in his family and peer groups,
at school and at work, and the leisure and recreational
facilities which are available in the community. Some
adolescents develop new coping skills as they meet the
demands of poor home, school and work environments. If
these attempts to cope are not successful, frustration is
experienced. Frustration is expressed in feelings which
range from irritation to extreme anger. It also results in
indirect forms of aggression. Frustration and stress are
also associated with the development of psychosomatic symptoms which include headaches, stomach upsets, sleep disturbance and body rashes (Ackerman, 1958). In prolonged
frustrating circumstances feelings of depression and apathy
are reported.

The second major emotional response to stress situations
is anxiety. High levels of anxiety are associated with feelings of inadequacy, loss of confidence, confusion in thinking
and, occasionally, panic. Severe anxiety is also expressed in the appearance of psychosomatic symptoms.

If stress situations are not reduced, and there is no increase in resources, the drain on the adolescent's emotional resources may be followed by exhaustion and a 'nervous
breakdown'. When stress situations cannot be modified
adolescents attempt to protect themselves by withdrawing
from them. Absenteeism from work and school is one of
the more obvious forms of withdrawal, but in more extreme
circumstances psychotic withdrawal may occur. Laing and
Esterson (1964), for instance, argue that it is stress within
the family which promotes schizophrenic disturbance, especially during late adolescence.

DEVELOPMENT DURING ADOLESCENCE

Having discussed some models of adolescence we now turn
to focus on development and behaviour during adolescence.
In discussing the changes which the adolescent has to face,
and the responses he and others make to these changes, we
continue to relate our discussion to the stress model. This
model would seem to be particularly useful for social workers who are having to decide how best to work with and for
an adolescent client, and the breadth of assessment which
the stress model offers can be related to the discussion in
Chapter three on the range and breadth of social work tasks
and social work practice. Table 2.2 presents a framework
which relates this stress model to some of the issues which
may arise in adolescent development.

Table 2.2 is based on a division of the adolescent's life
into four areas – the individual and personal aspects of
development (physical and sexual development, intellectual
and cognitive development, and emotional development);
group influences (primarily the family and the peer group);
the organisational context in which the adolescent spends
much of his time (especially the school and the work organisation); and, finally, community influences on the adolescent (such as the availability and use, or non-use, of
neighbourhood facilities, and the attitudes the wider community expresses towards the adolescent). The table also
notes some of the strengths and some of the weaknesses that
there may be for the adolescent in these differing areas of
functioning.

The stress model suggests that if a problem arises in one
area or arena of functioning we do not have to assume that
the resources to cope with that problem are also necessarily located within the same area of functioning. For example, conflict within the area of group functioning, such as
within the family or the peer group, may be met by resources and satisfactions within the organisational context of
the adolescent's life, such as success at school or satisfaction at work. This picture of an interrelating mesh of negative and positive influences on the adolescent is supported
by a major American study of adolescents who run away from
home. Brennan, Huizinga and Elliot (1978) studied a sample
of 800 self-reported runaways and a sample of 7,000 young
people who were representative of most young people.
They found that it was conflict within the home which usually
initially prompted young people to run away, but if the adol-

TABLE 2.2 A framework for understanding adolescent development

Problems (stress creation)	Resources (stress reduction)			
	Individual	Group	Organisation	Community
Individual early/late physical development emotional conflicts uncertain identity	Physical prowess; emotional stability; secure identity			
Group discord with parents delinquent peers rejection by peers		Supportive and authoritative parents; integrated and secure in peer group		
Organisation failure at school delinquent school anxious about schoolwork unsatisfying work unemployment unintegrated into work-group			Successful at school; belongs to caring school; satisfying employment; integrated into work group	
Community deprived neighbourhood rejection of youth and community facilities confusing and restricting legal status				Range of neighbourhood facilities; use of neighbourhood facilities; legal rights and protection

escent was having his needs for care and control, for success and satisfaction, met at school he would be unlikely to
run away despite conflict at home. However, if the adolescent was also involved with a delinquent peer group not only
would he be more likely to run away from home, but whilst
running away he would also be more likely to commit offences.

A particular difficulty for adolescents, and for the social
workers who may be involved with them, is that problems
and stresses tend to cluster so that the adolescent who is
in conflict with his parents is more likely to be involved
with a delinquent peer group, and he is also likely to be unsuccessful at school or to be unemployed. This interactional theme will emerge on several occasions during our
discussion of particular aspects of adolescent development,
but another theme will be that there often are compensatory
resources in an adolescent's life which can reduce the
impact of some of the stresses and conflicts which he, like
most other people, has to face. The task of the social
worker is to identify the stresses being experienced by the
adolescent and, whilst attempting to reduce these stresses
to identify and build on the strengths in the adolescent's
life. We now turn to look at some of these stresses and
problems and some of the strengths and resources.

ADOLESCENTS' STRESSES AND RESOURCES

The rapid growth spurt

Conger (1975) has stated that 'it is fair to say that adolescence begins in biology and ends in culture', and this
understanding of adolescence provides us with the logic for
our ordering of this discussion of some adolescent difficulties and possible solutions.

It is traditionally accepted that adolescence is that time
of life which is heralded by puberty, but that the onset of
puberty varies between generations and between individuals.
Puberty, as we have already noted, is the result of hormonal changes which lead to a relatively rapid burst in sexual
development and general body size, but not all aspects of
this development takes place at the same time or at the same
rate, and there is no necessary overriding sequence to this
development. Hence we need to be careful in assuming abnormality in development because one young person seems

to be out-of-step with his immediate peers. So what does happen during puberty?

One of the earliest indicators of puberty, which we briefly discussed in considering the constitutional model of development, is the 'growth spurt' which may start to occur for boys as early as $10\frac{1}{2}$ years, and for girls as early as $7\frac{1}{2}$ years (Conger, 1973). However, for the average boy the growth spurt is most pronounced between 13 and $15\frac{1}{2}$, and for the average girl the growth spurt is most pronounced between 11 and 13. The acceleration in stature can give added status to some adolescents, especially boys, who experience the growth spurt earlier as it adds to their physical superiority over their peers, but the growth spurt can also cause concern to many adolescents. For girls, for instance, there may be some embarrassment as they find themselves becoming taller than their friends as our cultural preference is that females should not be taller than men. There is also embarrassment for some adolescents as a result of their feeling awkward and out of control of their body. This may be because not all parts of the body grow at the same rate during the growth spurt. First the head, hands and feet grow rapidly, and this is followed by the accelerated growth of the arms and legs. Then body width increases before finally the trunk reaches its adult proportions. The adolescent may therefore feel and look uncoordinated and, at a time when young people are often concerned about their body image, he may feel uneasy with his physique.

The distressing consequence for those adolescents who come from financially deprived backgrounds is that they may find themselves wearing ill-fitting clothes – trousers may be too short, jackets too tight, or skirts too big. These adolescents will also often have a slower rate of development than their peers, as social class is associated with physical development. For example, a Home Office study of a sample of largely working-class 13-year-old approved school boys found that they were 'less tall, somewhat less heavy, but relatively less slender' than a comparative sample of London school boys (Field, Hammond and Tizard, 1971). This is partly explained by the changing dietary needs of adolescents to allow them to progress through the physical demands of the growth spurt. Sandstrom (1966) has stated that a man needs about 3,000 calories a day, but that a 13- to 16-year-old needs an extra 200 calories, and an older teenager needs about 3,800 calories. For females

the adult needs about 2,500 calories but the 13- to 15-
year-old needs another 300 calories. That a proportion of
adolescents have an unsatisfying diet partly accounts for
the finding of the National Child Development Study that 11
per cent of 16-year-olds are obese and another $12\frac{1}{2}$ per cent
are rated by doctors as thin (Fogelman, 1976a).

Sexual development

At the same time that the adolescent is having to adapt to a
changing body image he is also having to respond to his increasing sexuality. For boys the sequence of sexual
development is usually that the testes and scrotum enlarge,
that pubic hair grows, that the penis grows, there is a
growth of body and facial hair, and finally that the voice
deepens (Conger, 1973). For girls the sequence is an en-
largement (budding) of the breasts, the growth of pubic
hair, the growth of the vagina and the uterus, followed by
menarche. However, these aspects of sexual development
overlap and do not necessarily occur in this sequence.
    Findings from research concerning the implications of
early and late sexual maturation for boys shows that early
development of the signs of male maturity confers considerable advantages. These boys are reported to be more
self-confident and responsible and to show leadership
skills. Late maturing boys on the other hand are reported
to develop 'feelings of inadequacy and inferiority' (Lefrançois, 1976). For girls, Tanner (1962) has noted 'the
apparently inexplicable embarrassments of the girl who
menstruates earlier than anyone else or whose breasts grow
large while those of the remainder are still prepubertal'.
The late development of female sex characteristics may also
cause feelings of being very different from other girls.
The early or late development of breasts may have important
influences on an adolescent girl's awareness of her body,
i.e. her body image, and this is an integral part of her
physical self which is an important and sometimes crucial
aspect of her total identity. It has also been found that the
onset of menstruation has implications for the social status
of the girl amongst her peers. Faust (1960) collected data
from 731 girls in the USA and found that early and late
maturing girls (as measured by menarche) had low esteem
amongst same-age peers, but that girls who were in step
with the peer group's age of menstruation had high status.

So sexual maturation can be a source of status and
esteem, it can be a source of rejection and denigration by
peers if one is out of step with their development, and it
can also be a source of concern and anxiety if one has not
been adequately prepared and educated about sex and sexual
development.   Conflicts can occur about whether one is
developing normally and whether one is deviant in behaviour.   Masturbation, for instance, is often suspected to be
abnormal and disturbed, but research (Conger, 1973) has
shown that whereas only about 30 per cent of girls aged 20
state that they have ever masturbated, 92 per cent of 20-
year-old boys claim to have masturbated.

Intellectual development

Sexual development has implications for the emotional and
social functioning of the adolescent, and emotional and
social functioning are also related to the intellectual capabilities of the adolescent.   We need to distinguish between
IQ and mental ability.   As a general rule the scores from
IQ tests remain relatively stable during adolescence as the
tests allow for age differences in that one is measured
against the average for one's age group.   Mental ability
may, however, increase during adolescence as one acquires
increased skills in thinking and experiences qualitative
changes in one's intellectual performance.
Some adolescents do continue to improve their IQ, but
these are usually those adolescents who continue in full-
time education when many of their peers are no longer involved in education, and there is evidence that, because of
generational changes, adolescents are often more intelligent
than their parents (Conger, 1973).   This can be explained
by the greater educational opportunities available to adolescents compared to their parents.   But the major change in
intellectual functioning for most adolescents is qualitative
in that they have an increased ability to think abstractly.
As with physical and sexual development this change in intellectual capability occurs earlier for girls than for boys,
and there is also a sex difference in the areas of improved
intellectual functioning during adolescence.   Girls show a
greater improvement on measures of verbal ability whereas
boys show more improvement on measures of spatial ability.
This is probably due to differential social conditioning
rather than to any innate differences, as the sex differences

in intellectual ability are not noticeable in pre-school children.

Inhelder and Piaget (1958) have developed a stage theory of intellectual development which suggests that the determining characteristic of intellectual development for many adolescents is their new-found ability to think abstractly. They argue that existing, concrete reality no longer dominates thinking to the exclusion of other possibilities and that the adolescent has the ability to think about potential events and to question assumed wisdoms. This can lead to two possible consequences for the adolescent and for those who live with him. First, it can lead to an annoying and frustrating querying by the adolescent of the values of those around him, and by a propensity to seek and state ideal solutions to practical issues and problems. However, the idealism of adolescents is also seen by some commentators to be a positive source of social change: 'the first duty of youth is not to avoid mistakes but to show initiative and take responsibility, to make a tradition not to perpetuate one' (Tawney, quoted in Mays, 1965, p. i).

The second consequence for adolescents who are able to think more abstractly is that they may become more introspective. Not only do they question the statements and beliefs of others but they also question their own thoughts and developing ideology. This can be a confusing time when there may be no given or acceptable signposts to direct one's beliefs, but it can also be an exciting time of intellectual exploration and discovery. For some adolescents the journey progresses further than for others as their questioning is tolerated and even encouraged. This is particularly true of students. For other adolescents their questioning may be seen as confrontation, and they are discouraged and even penalised for challenging accepted wisdom.

Research by Adelson and O'Neil (1966) supports Piaget's theory that adolescents gradually develop the ability to think logically and hypothetically. In a study of 130 adolescents at ages 11, 13, 15 and 18 they found that younger adolescents are usually insensitive to individual liberties and opt for authoritarian solutions to political problems, but that as the adolescent gets older he makes greater use of philosophical principles in making political judgments. A similar picture emerged in later research by Adelson and O'Neil when they investigated the growth of the idea of law during adolescence:

Younger adolescents rarely imagined on their own – that
is, unless the interview item suggested it – that a law is
absurd, mistaken, or unfair. They assumed authority to
be omniscient and benign, hence law to be enacted only
for good and sufficient reasons.... By the time a child
is 15 – in some cases earlier – a very different tone of
discourse is evident. Now it is understood that law is a
human product, and that men are fallible; hence, law is
to be treated in the same sceptical spirit we treat other
human artifacts (Adelson, Green and O'Neil, 1969,
p. 332).
Hence during adolescence the individual may increase his
ability to think about alternative solutions to problems and
other responses to situations. He can speculate about the
consequences of his actions and can also more readily question the values and the norms of his society. This can be
seen as a resource for the adolescent who is now more able
to make decisions for himself on the basis of his own values
and beliefs, but it can also be a stressful time when those
around the adolescent are unwilling or unable to tolerate
his increasing assertiveness, or when the adolescent feels
confused himself about his own values and beliefs.

The family

Stress for the adolescent may be increased by pressures
within the family, but it is also true that for many adolescents the family is experienced as being supportive rather
than stressful. The stereotype of adolescence as a time of
identity crisis has been challenged,and the assumption that
adolescents are usually in conflict with their parents would
also seem to be incorrect. The portrayal of adolescence
as a time of conflict and crisis may be a reflection of the
bias in research to focus on the distressed, disturbed, or
delinquent teenager, and it may also reflect the attitude of
many adults to adolescents. For instance, it has been
argued (Musgrove, 1964; Pearson, 1978) that adolescents
have a more positive and tolerant attitude towards adults
than adults have towards young people. The supposed conflict with parents may also be due to the stress and identity
crisis felt by middle-aged parents rather than to any difficulties created by the adolescents (see Chapter five, and
Conger, 1973).
So what does research on adolescent–parent relationships

show?   The first conclusion to be drawn is that although
there will probably be occasional disagreements between
parents and adolescents there is rarely long-lasting conflict.   Rutter et al. (1976), in a major study of adolescents
on the Isle of Wight, found that although parents and adolescents often disagreed over issues such as dress and
length of hair there was very little evidence of parent-adolescent alienation at age 14.   Overt conflict between parents and adolescents was also found to be limited in the
National Child Development Study (Fogelman, 1976a) of
16,000 children.   This longitudinal study traced the development of all children born in one week in 1958 in Great
Britain.   When the children were aged 16 it was found that,
according to the parents, their relationships with their
children were very largely harmonious.   When conflict did
occur it was, as in Rutter's study, found to be about dress
or hairstyle, or the time of coming home at night and the
time of going to bed.   But even over these issues only 10
per cent of the parents said that they often disagreed with
their children.   A similar picture emerges from the statements of the adolescents.   Over 80 per cent stated that they
got on well with their mother, and 80 per cent also said that
they got on well with their father.   Very few (about 5 per
cent) said that they did not get on well with their parents.
A similar picture of a relative lack of adolescent-parent
disharmony is provided by Douvan and Adelson's (1966) research in America, and by Douglas (1967) in England and
Wales.
     The second conclusion to be drawn from the research on
adolescent-parent relationships is that parents remain a
major continuing influence on the adolescent.   The Isle of
Wight study concluded that:
     Parents continue to have a substantial influence on their
     children right through adolescence.   It is certainly true
     that peer group influences increase markedly during the
     teen-age period, but except in a minority of youngsters,
     they do not replace parental influences, although they
     sometimes rival them (Rutter, Graham, Chadwick and
     Yule, 1976, p. 54).
     The reviews of the relevant literature in Coleman (1978)
and in Cockram and Beloff (1978) present a good deal of
evidence to support the conclusion of Rutter and his colleagues, and it seems that parents continue throughout
adolescence to have a great deal of impact on the political,
moral and behavioural attitudes of their children (see also
Offer et al., 1970).

The third conclusion is that, although parents continue to
be a major influence in the adolescent's life, the adolescent
experiences some stress as he comes to spend more time
with his peers and gradually becomes more independent of
his parents. Rose and Marshall (1974) found, in their
study of the impact of school counsellors on the development
of adolescents in schools in Lancashire, that as the 'peer
orientation' and the amount of time spent with peers increa-
sed between the ages of $12\frac{1}{2}$ to $14\frac{1}{2}$, the 'home orientation'
of the adolescents decreased while the 'home relations
worry' score increased. This was especially true for
boys (this reflects the greater move away from home by
boys compared to girls). Hence an increase in orientation
towards peers leads to some difficulties at home and to increased anxiety about relationships with parents. This
finding is also supported by Coleman's research (1974) on
the focal concerns of adolescents. He found that relationships with parents were a positive theme for both boys and
girls at age 11, but that later in mid-adolescence relationships with parents led to anxiety. Coleman, like Rose and
Marshall, also identifies sex differences in relationships
with parents:

> Conflict with parents, it appears, starts earlier and ends
> earlier for girls. Even more significant than this, how-
> ever, is the fact that the conflict revolves around differ-
> ent issues, which may be the reason for the slightly dif-
> ferent time course. For boys the conflict is to do with
> independence of action, freedom of movement, true behav-
> ioural autonomy. Girls on the contrary do not indicate
> this to be an issue. They rarely express themes of
> direct conflict, but are much more frequently concerned
> with inner autonomy. Girls want to be able to be them-
> selves. They feel threatened, sometimes even over-
> whelmed, by the influence and forcefulness of their
> parents, and they are clearly anxious that they will not
> be allowed to be the person they want to be. This is
> where the conflict lies for them (Coleman, 1974, p. 142).

The fourth conclusion to be drawn from the research on
parent-adolescent relationships is that there are differential relationships between adolescents and their mothers and
their fathers. Willmott (1966) in his study of 246 working-
class boys in East London, found that mothers were seen as
more understanding than fathers and that this was because
'the strains over authority within the immediate family make
it difficult for adolescent boys and their fathers to be at

ease' (Willmott, 1966, p. 72). The proportion of parents seen as 'very understanding' varied during adolescence, as is shown in Figure 2.1.

Age of adolescents

14	15	16	17	18	19	20

Mum   ◄–52%–►   ◄–––– 42% –––––►   ◄–61%–►

Dad   ◄–43%–►   ◄––––– 36% ––––––►   ◄–34%–►

FIGURE 2.1 Perceptions of parents as very understanding

This picture of possible conflict with fathers for a proportion of adolescents is also reflected in a major study of detached youth work where social workers were used to contact 'at risk' adolescents in the community. The workers found that 'the (adolescents) use of leisure was very much influenced by the need to get out of the home and away from their fathers' (Smith, Farrant and Marchant, 1972, p. 91). However, it may need stressing again that for the majority of adolescents their relationships with their parents are more harmonious than conflict-ridden, despite the occasional transitory mutual irritation.

For girls there is some rather dated evidence that in their relationships with their mothers they experience more conflict than in their relationships with their fathers (Liccione, 1955). The peak age for this conflict was 15 and it was seen to arise because it was the mothers who were primarily and immediately responsible for controlling and restricting the behaviour of the girls, but this finding is not supported by more recent research (Rose and Marshall, 1974):

> The move of girls away from home appears to be somewhat less drastic ... and does not affect their relationship with their mothers appreciably. In line with this, their home relations scores do not increase significantly.

There are, however, families in which particular difficulties seem to arise or become more pronounced during adolescence. For single parent families, for instance, there are problems of one parent (usually the mother who has only a small income) being unable to offer the child all the opportunities she would like to offer (Ferri and Robinson, 1976), being unable to offer adequate control and supervision (Marsden, 1973) and not being able to share in all the interests of the adolescent because these interests

(e.g. watching soccer) are seen to be related to the roles
and interests of only one sex (Ferri and Robinson, 1976).
This is not to say that children from single parent families
necessarily experience more conflict with their parents
than other adolescents, but they are more likely to experience deprivation and lack of opportunity during their childhood and adolescence which may create strains on their
relationships with their parents.

It is also now well documented that the quality of parenting is associated with delinquency during adolescence.
For instance, in the Institute of Criminology's longitudinal
study of over 400 boys from 'a typical working-class urban
neighbourhood' in London it was found that poor parenting
was related to delinquency:

> The poor parental behaviour factor was a global impres-
> sion of family conflict and generally unsatisfactory paren-
> tal attitude and discipline, taking into account both the
> emotional quality and the techniques of child-rearing.
> Parental behaviour was shown to have an important influ-
> ence upon the likelihood of delinquency, independently of
> social factors such as low income and large family.
> These results lend strong support to the theory that the
> unsatisfactory attitudes and methods of individual parents
> play an important part in the genesis of juvenile delin-
> quency, over and above the influence of external social
> pressures (West and Farrington, 1973, p. 192).

There is a good deal of evidence that many delinquents
and other adolescents who are underachieving at school
have especially poor relationships with their fathers
(Andry, 1960; Mack, 1976; Lambert and Hart, 1976;
Smith and Walters, 1978), and West and Farrington (1973)
in the study quoted above also found that poor parental
supervision, which was defined as 'a lack of watchfulness
(vigilance) over the boy's activities and a lack of concern
with the enforcing of rules', was associated with delinquency. This conclusion is supported by Wilson's (1974) research in the Midlands. She found that 'chaperonage' by
parents was the most effective way of stopping those adolescents who lived in some neighbourhoods from becoming involved in delinquency. However, the difficulty which some
parents will have in offering this chaperonage is highlighted
in Parker's (1974) study of adolescents in Liverpool:

> The mother of a typically Roundhouse family, tied to the
> baby of the moment, simply could not cope, in her small,
> often grossly overcrowded, badly sound-proofed flat, if

she kept all the kids indoors. There is no garden, no organised and supervised play space, not even a back yard. The flat is above ground level, and once inside the door the children are on a narrow landing which is a thoroughfare to passageways, corners, stairs and freedom. Kids will demand to play out, mother has no option and the saga begins. Over the months and years it becomes standard practice for little Tommy to disappear 'out' for most of his free time. As the infant gets to school age, mother returns to work - if she ever gave it up: she is likely to be a waitress, day or night, or perhaps a sales assistant or an office cleaner. She will be unable to look after the kids during the holidays, she will be tired when she is at home. Since working is necessary if ends are to meet, nearly all mums undertake it accepting it as normal. The kids consequently have very free, unrestricted and exploratory childhoods (Parker, 1974, p. 40).

However, following the findings of West and Farrington and of Wilson, it may need stressing that supervision and the enforcement of rules does not mean that harsh physical punishment is desirable. Although there are class differences in styles of punishing children (Newsom and Newsom, 1963 and 1968), even within a social class there is evidence that a cluster of factors which includes a reliance on physical punishment is related to delinquency. West (1967, p. 76), and Conger (1973) compare 'authoritative' parenting with 'authoritarian' and 'permissive' parenting. 'Authoritative' parenting occurs when the parent assumes ultimate responsibility for the adolescent but still values the adolescent's self-will and self-motivated disciplined behaviour. Their exercise of parental authority is based on explanation and discussion with the adolescent. 'Authoritarian' parenting is based on the unexplained and often intolerant imposition of the parent's will, and 'permissive' parenting can be characterised as an abdication of parental responsibility for the adolescent. Conger suggests that it is 'authoritative' parenting which leads to the adolescent becoming a mature, self-reliant adult. The adolescent who is the subject of 'authoritarian' parenting is more likely to be in conflict with his parents.

A set of adolescents who may be more likely to be in conflict with their parents are immigrants where the culture of the parents is in conflict with the indigenous youth culture, or where the adolescents see the parents' culture as

being out of touch with the realities that they are having to
face (Ford, 1975). For instance, West Indian adolescents
seem to have particular demands made on them by their
parents to be successful at school and at work, and these
demands are in conflict with the limited opportunities and
the discrimination which the adolescents experience (Mack,
1977). The adolescents respond to this cultural conflict
and the stress that it creates by increasing their involvement with the peer group. Their behaviour may be in conflict with the behaviour demanded by other groups in the
community and by their parents, and the adolescents may
explicitly set themselves apart from the other groups to
show that they reject the social values of others as much as
they are rejected by them ... their response becomes pro-
active rather than reactive. The ideology of these adolescents and young people may not be fully developed, but their
attitudes become more decisive and explicit (see Philips,
1976; Pryce, 1979).

The peer group

The suggestion in our discussion on the parent-adolescent
relationship in many West Indian families in Britain is that
adolescents may increase their orientation to the peer
group partly as a result of pressures from within the
family. There is evidence that some adolescents may be
'pushed' into a dependency on the peer group by their
parents even more than they are 'pulled' into this allegiance
by peer group pressures (Bowerman and Kinch, 1959;
Smith, 1974), and this can also be related to the comment
quoted earlier from the Wincroft Youth Project (Smith, Farrant and Marchant, 1972) that many of the unattached youth
with whom they had contact spent time away from home because of conflict with their fathers. In another study of
detached youth work with girls (Marchant and Smith, 1977)
it was found that 25 of their sample of 27 girls experienced
stress at home but that only 16 of the 25 were seen to contribute to this stress. The girls involved in this project
were at risk in many ways:
> poor attendance at school or employment, stress at home
> and staying away from home overnight, association with
> delinquents, roughs and gypsies, inadequate social con-
> tacts, inadequate social behaviour, involvement with
> drugs and attention-seeking appearance (Farrant and
> Smith, 1977, p. 77).

Hence the picture which emerges is that it is too simple to say that adolescents increase their allegiance to the peer group just because the peer group provides excitement and fun, as we also need to be aware of the other pressures which might predispose an adolescent to a greater degree of peer group allegiance.

We also need to recognise the pressures that the peer group creates for the adolescent. Coleman, in his study of 347 boys and 392 girls attending public, grammar and secondary schools in south east England, found that relationships with the peer group remained major focal concerns for young people during their secondary schooling, but that the content of these concerns changed during adolescence. Table 2.3, which is reproduced from Coleman (1974, p. 137), shows how the adolescents' concerns about the peer group changed, and the table also notes changes in the adolescent's attitude to parents and to himself.

Table 2.3 shows that for both boys and girls at age 11 relationships with parents and authority in large group settings are seen positively by the adolescent. However, being on one's own, and relationships with the opposite sex are a cause of some anxiety for them. By age 15, however, heterosexual relationships are seen positively by both boys and girls, but relationships within the peer group are a source of some anxiety, although the content of this anxiety varies between the sexes:

FRIENDSHIP. Where negative themes are concerned girls express a significantly greater proportion which indicate fears of rejection in the three person situation. REJECTION IN THE LARGE GROUP. With regard to this issue girls express more themes which imply an identification with the individual, while boys express a greater number indicating group identification (Coleman, 1974, p. 141).

Therefore, although adolescents may come to spend an increasing amount of time with their peers during mid-adolescence (Rose and Marshall, 1974; Willmott, 1966), the peer group is not necessarily an anxiety-free, safe haven for them but rather it creates in its own right many stresses and conflicts for the adolescent (Douvan and Adelson, 1966).

This is of particular relevance to much social work with adolescents. For example, in an intermediate treatment group which was studied by one of us there were two girls who were isolated from, and taunted by, the main group of five girls. One of these stopped attending the group, but

TABLE 2.3 The focal concerns of adolescents (from Coleman, 1974)

Age	BOYS Constructive	BOYS Negative	GIRLS Constructive	GIRLS Negative
11	parental relationship authority in large group	solitude heterosexual relationship	parental relationship authority in large group	solitude heterosexual relationship
13				
15	heterosexual relationship	friendship in small group rejection from large group	heterosexual relationship	parental relationship friendship in small group rejection from large group
17	solitude rejection from large group	internal conflict over future identity authority in large group	solitude rejection from large group	internal conflict over future identity authority in large group

the other continued to attend.   She had no friends outside
the group and the group provided her with one of her very
limited experiences of peer group activity outside the school
classroom.   This girl was bullied and teased by some of the
other girls in the group, and after she became upset and
cried because she was being teased she did not attend the
group the following week.   This caused a great deal of concern to the other girls, who were embarrassed that they had
teased her, and were distressed that she had become upset
and had now missed attending.   This led to some discussion
and the girls decided that two of them would call to see her
to apologise and to ask her to come to the group again.
They visited her at home and the girl did continue to attend
the group.   This was probably an important experience for
her as here were her peers asking her to join them again.
It was also probably a significant experience for the other
girls who had, reflecting Coleman's finding, become distressed about one girl being isolated within a small group
but who had then taken some self-motivated action to rectify
this.

Coleman's research also found, however, that by the time
adolescents are leaving school they change their orientation
towards the peer group.   They are concerned about being
controlled in large groups, and dislike this control, and
they are beginning to feel that independence from the peer
group is positive and desirable.   This does not mean that
peer group activity ceases, but that it changes in style and
meaning for the adolescent.   For instance, rather than
larger single sex groupings being the predominant form of
peer group, smaller heterosexual groupings develop (see
Chapter six).   This leads to heterosexual pairing and Willmott (1966), for example, found that whereas 14- and 15-
year-old boys had 'little to do with girls', between ages 16
and 18 most of the boys were 'taking girls out sometimes',
and by ages nineteen and twenty 'more than a quarter' of his
sample of working-class boys were engaged.

The impression may exist that the peer group is a relatively structured and consistent entity rather than a contin-
ually changing and fluctuating gathering.   Indeed on the
continuum of gang-group-gathering it may be that much of
the activity of adolescents takes place in loosely structured
gatherings rather than in consistent groupings or highly
structured gangs.   This was found to be so by Gill in his
participant observation research of adolescents on the
street corner in one neighbourhood of a northern city:

This group was not however a constant grouping over time
and friendship patterns in Luke Street as elsewhere were
not static; thus in some ways the collective name of the
'boys on Casey's corner' makes the group appear more
homogenous, more defined, and more constant than it
actually was. In fact the group was composed of small
groups or pairs of friends, and although an individual
boy would know all the others who 'knocked around on the
corner' he might only have close contact with two or three
of them (Gill, 1977, p. 98).

There is also often a common assumption that the peer
group becomes the determining influence on the adolescents'
behaviour and attitudes, but this view has been challenged.
First, as we have discussed above, parents still have a
major influence on the adolescent. For instance, in Coleman's (1961) research on adolescents in America, 70 per
cent of his large sample stated that they would not join a
club if their parents disapproved, and Conger writes that:

neither parental nor peer influence is monolithic, extending to all areas of adolescent decision-making and behaviour. The weight given to either parental or peer opinion depends to a significant degree on the adolescent's
appraisal of its relative value in a specific situation.
For example, peer influence is more likely to be predominant in such matters as tastes in music and entertainment,
fashions in clothing and language, patterns of same- and
opposite-sex peer interaction, and the like. Parental
influence is more likely to be predominant in such areas
as underlying moral and social values, and understanding
of the adult world (Conger, 1973, p. 291).

This echoes the findings of the National Child Development
Study (Fogelman, 1976a), which we have already quoted,
that disagreements between parents and adolescents, when
they occurred, were usually around issues of hairstyle,
dress, and time of coming home and going to bed at night.
However, unlike Conger's statement, the National Child Development Study found little disagreement (3 per cent) between
parents and adolescents over the friendship choices of the
adolescents.

There is also evidence that adolescents, and especially
older adolescents, are not necessarily determined in their
actions by the peer group, regardless of parental influence. For instance, Landbaum and Willis (1971) found that
younger adolescents were much more conforming to the
opinions of high status members of their peer group than

were older adolescents, and this can be related to Coleman's (1974) finding that independence from the peer group, and being able to make decisions oneself rather than following the party line, are seen as positive attributes by the 17-year-old. However, as Conger has written (1973, p. 305):

> to expect the average adolescent - unsure of his own identity and unclear about the demands that will be made upon him in a confused, rapidly changing society - to be immune to the favour of his peers would be unrealistic and inappropriate. Most adolescents, at one time or another, feel that they do not belong, and the pain, however temporary, can be very real.

This may help us to understand the difficult and delinquent peer group motivated behaviour which is exhibited by some adolescents at school and during their leisure.

The school

The National Child Development Study (Fogelman, 1976a) found that only 11 per cent of their sample saw school as a waste of time, although 30 per cent stated that they did not like school. However many of the adolescents who are in contact with social workers are in difficulties at school and they create difficulties for teachers. Hargreaves (1967), in his participant observation study of a secondary school, traces how some pupils gradually increase their commitment to the school during the years of secondary education whereas others became more alienated from the school regime. This may be due to parental attitudes (Marsden and Jackson, 1966) which see education as remote and possibly irrelevant, but it may also be due to processes operating within the school. Hargreaves found in his study that those in lower streams, who saw themselves as having very few opportunities for success in school, became more disruptive of classes, and that status within their friendship groups was allied to their challenging and confrontational risk-taking behaviour. For those in the academically-achieving higher streams, however, peer group status was associated with working hard and being successful in one's work. The peer group, therefore, can be seen to be responding to, as well as creating, stresses and successes within the school. This scenario is supported by the more impressionistic writings of Willis (1978) and Corrigan (1979) who found that

some pupils see teachers as unfair and inconsistent in
their attitudes, and these adolescents see schooling as more
about control than about education. The attitudes of these
pupils is understandable when it is related to Hargreaves'
(1975) research on deviance in classrooms and how teacher-
pupil interactions may only serve to heighten and confirm
deviance.

In this context there is also some evidence that some
schools may actually promote delinquency, poor attendance
and low academic attainment (Power, 1967; Reynolds, 1976;
Rutter, 1979), and it is suggested that rigid streaming by
ability, high rates of corporal punishment, high staff turn-
over, and a custodial or authoritarian school climate are
key factors in delinquency-promoting schools (Reynolds and
Jones, 1978). However good schools can also have a positive influence on children, and can compensate for some
deficiencies in other areas of the child's life. For example, Douglas (1967),in his longitudinal study of over 4,000
children born in 1946, found that:

> It seems that good teaching in primary schools can make
> up for deficiencies in parental interest, so that, in the
> schools with the best record of grammar school awards,
> the children whose parents take little interest in their
> school progress do as well as those whose parents take
> much interest (Douglas, 1967, p. 143).

However, when severe 'social handicap' (a measure composed of social class, family size, adequacy of children's
clothing, and parental contact with school) is present,
schools seem unable to compensate for disadvantage in other
areas of a child's life (Wilson and Herbert, 1974).

Leisure

Following the time the adolescent spends at home with his
family and the time he spends at school (or at work), it is
leisure time that accounts for the third major activity area
of his life. We have already noted that during adolescence
young people spend an increasing amount of time away from
their parents, and this time is usually spent in the company
of their peers. For many young people a proportion of this
time is spent in organised and supervised activity, like
attendance at youth clubs or involvement in structured sport-
ing activities. A study by the Office of Population Censuses
and Surveys (1969) found that 72 per cent of boys and 58 per

cent of girls were attached to some form of club, and that 93
per cent had been involved with a club at some stage.   Factors such as social class and the geographical location of
the club affect the club's membership, and there is evidence
that young people from middle-class homes are more likely
to be members of many clubs and to be actively involved in
committee work and decision making within youth clubs
(Eggleston, 1975).   This picture can be related to the
social patterns of the areas in which the adolescents live:

> The data were then examined for any relationship between
> the social status of the individual and committee member-
> ship within the clubs.   Overall, 30 per cent of the chil-
> dren of manual workers and 40 per cent of the children of
> non-manual workers showed little interest in the club
> committee.   However, when the position within the club
> was examined, it appeared that in the predominantly
> middle class club, Uptown Grammar, no children of
> manual workers were either on the committee or wished
> to be on it.   This was also reflected, to some extent, in
> Colourview Rise.   When the attitudes of the members of
> the traditional working class club (Colliery Bank) and the
> club in the culturally deprived area (Coronation Estate)
> are considered together the picture is strikingly differ-
> ent.   Though their social composition is similar, 50 per
> cent in the traditional working class area as opposed to
> 21 per cent in the deprived area would like to be on the
> committee.   The latter follows the expected pattern, the
> former is markedly different.   It is difficult to suggest
> reasons for this but the local significance of the branch
> committee of the National Union of Mineworkers, particu-
> larly at the time of the survey when a major national
> strike was taking place, may have some importance
> (Eggleston, 1975, p. 109).

The suggestion from Eggleston's research is that the behaviour and attitudes of the adolescents reflects the attitudes
of the parent community in which they live, and here again
we have evidence of the continuing influence of parental
values and expectations on adolescents and their use of
leisure.

For many of the adolescents in contact with social workers, however, there is evidence that they are not attending,
or have only limited involvement with, youth clubs.   Davies
(1969) found that over a third of his sample of 462 male probationers aged between 17 and 20 had never attended a
youth club, that a quarter of those who had attended a youth

club had not done so for at least 6 months, and that only just over a fifth had attended a youth club within the previous month. Davies found that:

> At all times (during the last weekend) except Sunday morning, a majority of the men went out: looked at from another direction, however, it may be found surprising that as many as a quarter stayed in on a Saturday evening, a third on a Sunday evening, and almost half on Sunday afternoon ... just over a quarter of the probationers (27.3%) spent the weekend almost wholly within the home setting, mixing only with their parents or siblings, while slightly under a half (44.8%) were out of the house most of the time and in the company of people other than their immediate relations (Davies, 1969, p. 191).

Although a sizeable proportion of Davies's sample of probationers seemed more home-centred than might have been anticipated, the overriding impression is that adolescents and young people who get into trouble are, not surprisingly, those who spend their leisure time away from home. Much of this time is spent in unstructured and unsupervised activity, as West (1977) found in his follow-up study of 389 working-class young men when they were aged 18:

> judging by middle-class standards, the use of leisure by many of the Study youths might be described as somewhat haphazard, disorganised and generally unconstructive. Home hobbies, reading and attending youth clubs or evening classes were not popular. Delinquents, compared with non-delinquents, spent more time away from home, sometimes aimlessly riding around or hanging about in the street (although this was often an euphemism for looking for girls), but more frequently in locations such as pubs, discotheques and parties (West and Farrington, 1977, p. 70).

However, for younger adolescents many of these leisure resources (the pub, the discotheque, and even some youth clubs and, at some times, the cinema) are not available or accessible, and their use of leisure is partly determined by this availability.

Hence, the National Child Development Study (Fogelman, 1976a) found that many 16-year-olds are dissatisfied with the amenities available to them in their neighbourhood. However, the same National Child Development Study found that at age 11 the boredom experienced by their sample was not related to the lack of local amenities (Fogelman, 1976b).

About a third of the 11-year-olds claimed that they always enjoyed their spare time, about two-thirds stated that they sometimes got bored, and only about 3 per cent claimed that they often got bored. At age 11 boredom was not found to be related to delinquency, poor local facilities, or to tele-vision watching. It was however, found to be related to less able children, lower social class, large families, little paternal interest, and to a less varied use of leisure time.

The picture which emerges, therefore, is that those chil-dren who may be experiencing more difficulties and fewer opportunities at home, and who are less able, are least likely to make full use of the leisure amenities and opportu-nities which are available to them locally. The suggestion is that those who may have the greatest need for a range of leisure opportunities to compensate for the stresses, diffi-culties and deprivations in the home are also those who are least likely to make use of these resources and opportuni-ties, even when they are available. Stress in one area of one's life makes it more difficult to take advantage of com-pensatory resources in other areas.

This picture is reflected in much of the writings on adol-escent street-corner culture. The activities of young people out on the street may lead them into trouble as they attempt to create some excitement in an otherwise drab and boring environment (Parker, 1974; Gill, 1977; Corrigan, 1979). These are often the adolescents who are not suc-cessful at school and who are in conflict at home. They are not integrated into youth service provision and they are likely to be unemployed or to be in unstimulating, low-status jobs (Willis, 1978). The street-corner peer group provides one of their limited sources of fun and acceptance (for a humourous novelistic account of the street-corner peer group see Bleasdale, 1975). However, much of the time on the street corner is spent 'dossing around', and even when the adolescents are not involved in law breaking (such as vandalism and theft) they may still be seen as a disturbance and a threat. They may be arrested on 'sus' or they may be moved on by the police. It is these confrontations with the police which are seen to lead to, and to reflect, the labelling of adolescents as delinquent within the neighbour-hood (Gill, 1976).

Youth styles

The perception of these adolescents as delinquent and as a disturbance is heightened by their ostentatious style of dress and attitude (see S. Cohen, 1972). Each generation of young people seem, not surprisingly, to want to establish their own particular identity and style, but this is often interpreted as deviant and as a threat by the adult community. The style of young people, and especially the cult styles developed by working-class adolescents, are seen as bizarre and ridiculous by many adults, but it is possible to locate the genesis of the styles within their parent cultures and to relate them to contemporary cultural concerns. Whether it be the Teds, the Mods and the Rockers, the Skinheads or the Punks, their dress and their attitudes can be linked to the concerns of their time and their class.

Clarke and Jefferson (1976) define style as: 'the result of a process of appropriation of disparate objects and symbols from their normal social context and their reworking by members of the group into a new and coherent whole with its own special significance' (Clarke and Jefferson, 1976, p. 152), and the Skinheads, for example, took traditional styles of working men's dress and emphasised their distinctive features: 'The clothes, heavy denims, plain or striped button-down shirts, braces and heavy boots, created an image which was clean-cut, smart and functional – a youthful version of working clothes' (Clarke and Jefferson, 1976, p. 156).

The attitudes of the Skinheads also reflected working-class concerns. The emphasis on masculinity and on being tough (as in 'queer-bashing'), the scape-goating and victimisation of Asian immigrants ('Paki-bashing'), the working-class puritanism about the work ethic, and the stressing of territory and one's own neighbourhood (reflected, for instance, in 'holding your own end' at soccer grounds, see Marsh, 1978, and Taylor, 1971) are all adaptations and exaggerations of traditional working-class concerns: 'In the skinhead style we can see both the elements of continuity (in terms of the style's content), and discontinuity (in terms of its form), between parent culture and youth sub-culture' (Clarke, 1975, p. 102).

It is also possible to link the genesis of styles to each other (see P. Cohen, 1972) and to see how there is historical continuity between styles – one style often developing in opposition to the focal concerns predominant within the

preceding style and each style also reflecting the changing
social attitudes and economic and employment conditions of
its time.   The Skinheads reflected a time in the late 1960s
and early 1970s when the 'never had it so good' 1950s were
giving way to the recession of the 1970s.   Unemployment
was increasing and liberal social attitudes and values were
giving way to the reactionary and conservative focus on
social control and competition.   'Lame ducks' and 'scroun-
gers' replaced the 'love and peace' and 'do your own thing'
slogans of the 1960s.   People began to dig themselves in
for the hard time to come.

Therefore far from youth styles being incomprehensible
and senseless, they can be seen as extending and emphasising concerns and attitudes within their parent culture.
Rather than representing counter-cultures or unrelated
subcultures, they have their roots in contemporary cultural
and class issues.   They reflect the stresses, strains and
contradictions within society and within the parent culture.
They are also vulnerable to exploitation, especially by the
mass media, who either cast young people as 'folk devils'
(S. Cohen, 1972) to be consumed by an adult market, or who
see adolescents as a consumer market in their own right:

  it is our contention, therefore, that changes in working
  class youth culture are, in an important sense, manufac-
  tured changes, imposed on the mass via the media, and
  determined primarily by sales potential ... in circumstances where the cultural domination is economically
  determined by a consumer industry, the cultural innova-
  tions will be both circumscribed and distorted by the
  marketing initiatives and strategies necessarily engaged
  in by the agents of consumerism (Taylor and Wall, 1976,
  p. 120).

Money and work

As Abrams found in his study on teenage spending in the
1950s:

  the teenage market is almost entirely working class.
  Its middle class members are either still at school and
  college or else only just beginning on their careers: in
  either case they dispose of much smaller incomes than
  their working class contemporaries and it is highly probable, therefore, that not far short of 90 per cent of all
  teenage spending is conditioned by working class taste
  and values (Abrams, 1959, p. 13).

This is a view which is supported by Eggleston's (1975) research on youth club members. He found that the members
of the youth clubs located in working-class areas had more
money to spend than those who came from middle-class
areas, and that this was related to their earning powers.

However, for those adolescents still at school their
opportunity to earn money is severely limited. The National Child Development Study (Fogelman, 1976a) found that
about a quarter of their sample of 16-year-olds had some
part-time employment, but that only about a third of these
earned more than £3 a week. When asked about the pocket
money which they were given just under a half were receiving no more than £1 a week. For many it is the promise of a wage packet and money in the pocket that provides
an incentive to leave school at the earliest opportunity:

There was almost no mention at all of the process of work
itself as an important reason for leaving school; rather,
most of those who mentioned work as a reason specified
the rewards of work, and this in a very specific way ...
the concrete results of getting a job when you leave
school are those that can be imagined at the time - namely, more money in your pocket to spend in the way in
which you spend it now (Corrigan, 1979, p. 75).

However the transition from school to work is not an easy
one for many adolescents. Today a large number are leaving school with the prospect of unemployment, the dole
queue and boredom rather than the promise of a job. For
them adult status also brings 'scrounger' status, and in an
attempt to counter this process a range of interim employment opportunities was introduced (Job Creation, Step,
etc.). But even for those who do find a job on leaving
school the transition from pupil to employee is not without
its strains and stresses:

In the sociological perspective (going to work) is probably as overwhelmingly important as the onset of puberty
is biologically and psychologically. There is something
very definite about leaving school. It is, in a very real
sense, the end of true childhood (Mays, 1972, p. 249).

Mays argues that in the year before leaving school the
adolescent has to face 'a period of stressful anxiety' about
his future, and that this stress goes some way to explain
why the year prior to the school leaving age shows a peak
in the incidence of delinquency - the delinquency is seen as
a reaction to this stress. Mays also argues that after
being in work for a few years the older adolescent has to

face another period of 'psychological difficulty' when he
comes to realise that, without training or qualifications,
he is destined to spend the next fifty years in unsatisfying
labour for limited financial reward.   This, according to
Mays, accounts for much of the delinquency of older adolescents.   There is some evidence from Willmott (1966) that
although Mays's explanation of delinquency is rather limited
in its range, young school leavers do experience this crisis
of work identity.   Willmott found that at a time when the
school leaving age was 15 'relatively few' of his 15- and
16-year-old working-class boys were dissatisfied with
work and that this was also true of 19- and 20-year-olds.
However, at ages 17 and 18 there were many more boys who
were discontented with their employment.   Possibly this
goes some way to account for Davies's (1969) findings that
40.9 per cent of his sample of 17- to 20-year-old probationers had unsteady work records and only 26.8 per cent
had steady work records.   Davies (1974) found that employment was a focus in interviews between probation officers and probationers in 52 per cent of cases, which gives
some measure of the importance attached to employment,
and the difficulties seen to be created by unemployment, by
probation officers.   Their concern is supported by Davies's
(1969) finding that those probationers who had poor employment records were those most likely to re-offend within one
year of the making of the probation officer.   There would,
therefore, seem to be some relationship, although not necessarily a causal link, between unemployment (or unsteady
employment) and law breaking (see also Gladstone, 1979).

The law

Our final comments on understanding adolescents marks the
end of our exploration of adolescence - we started by focusing on the physiological changes which herald and accompany
adolescence and we end by looking at those special changes
in social status which also face the adolescent.   There is
a confusing range of legislation which relates particularly
to adolescents and which signifies their gradual entry into
adult rights and responsibilities.   At times society seems
to be saying to the adolescent that they are and should be
adult, but at other times society's formal laws confirm the
adolescent's continuing child status.   Table 2.4 records
some of the ages limits within legislation.

TABLE 2.4 Legal age limits and the adolescent

Age	
10	Age of criminal responsibility
13	Below this age (with a few exceptions) children cannot be employed
14	Below 14 boys cannot be found guilty of rape Can be sent to a detention centre Can be issued with certain types of firearm certificate Can see a film with an AA certificate Can go into licensed premises, but cannot drink alcohol while there
15	Can be sent to borstal
16	Can leave school Girl can legally consent to sexual intercourse May be eligible for supplementary benefit Boys may join the armed forces (girls must be aged 17) Can apply for legal aid May marry (in England and Wales parental consent is required until 18)
17	Can be given a prison sentence
18	Eligible to vote Can choose where to live May watch a film with an X certificate May drink alcohol in a pub May enter a betting shop
21	May adopt Male homosexual acts legal in private (no law on female homosexuality)

The picture which emerges from this partial exploration of the law and adolescents is that adolescence is a time when society sometimes seems as confused about the adolescent as the adolescent is presumed to be confused about society.

SUMMARY

This chapter has explored some explanations of adolescent behaviour. It has discussed in detail a stress model of the interaction between adolescent problems and the resources which social workers can seek to develop to help their clients cope with these problems.

The first area of concern to be discussed was the rapid growth spurt and attention was directed towards the wide range of individual differences in the age of onset of puberty. It was noted that earlier or later development of the rapid growth spurt can cause considerable anxiety for the adolescent. Sexual development was also found to be a source of some apprehension. Intellectual development can also cause problems for those young people who turn to think in abstract rather than concrete terms. These new ways of thinking may stimulate them to challenge 'the conventional wisdom of experience' which older people may use to solve their problems.

The fourth area of possible problems and resources to be considered was the families of adolescents. Little research support was found for the proposition that contemporary youth finds it very difficult to communicate with their parents. It was suggested that contrary to popular belief our conclusion is that parents remain an important influence in the lives of their sons and daughters, though this framework of guidance and support weakens as the peer group becomes a major frame of reference for adolescents. Three styles of parenting were discussed (i.e. authoritative, authoritarian and permissive) and the problems which the last two of these generated were reported. One response to these problems is a strong identification which the peer group though it is sometimes a case of jumping from the frying pan of family conflict into the fire of severe pressures to conform to peer group norms of behaviour, dress, values and language. Later, there is likely to be a development of a relationship with a boy friend or girl friend. It is these relationships which can become major areas of support for the older adolescent.

For the younger adolescent the focus of peer group relationships is the school, and for boys and girls in middle adolescence it is the youth club and the neighbourhood which provides a major venue for the peer group. Many of them complain of limited leisure facilities, but there is evidence to indicate that they may have few of the social skills needed to use these resources. For a number of adolescents their responses to these problems is to develop life-styles which include aggressive behaviour, racial intolerance and political extremism such as membership of the National Front (see Robins and Cohen, 1978). The demands on adolescents also include the transition from school to work, though an increasing number have to cope with the pressures of unemployment. Finally we commented on the law in relation to adolescents and we found a conflicting range of legislative status for the adolescent, which is probably confusing to many adolescents and their parents.

In our stress framework for understanding the different problems which have to be faced in society we have also delineated some of the resources which can be developed at the individual, group, organisation and community levels. We have reported the importance of the support of 'authoritative' parents and of caring schools, and we have indicated the necessity of adolescents learning the skills to make maximum use of the available community facilities. It is the social worker's task to minimise the stresses which impinge on their adolescent clients, and to increase utilisation of the available resources.

Chapter three

The relevance of unitary
models in social work
with adolescents

Florence Rossetti

/Following the discussion in Chapter two of some models of
adolescence, and the exploration of the personal and social
development of young people, Rossetti turns to examine
social work theory and method. This paper considers the
problem of how to conceptualise social work so as to encompass the individual and the social environment, in the interests of effective assessment and help, across the whole
range of social work practice. There is a discussion of a
dynamic conceptualisation of social work, based upon a
systems paradigm, and a focus on unitary models of practice, which allow the adolescent to be located within his
social context. The chapter also seeks to provoke thought
about the validity of the traditional forms of social work
being considered as integral methods in their own right.
The paper therefore offers a framework and an argument
against which the later intervention contributions can be
considered./

INTRODUCTION

The central focus of social work has long been claimed to
be the client-in-his-situation, the interaction of individuals
with their social environment. The implication has been
that both the problem for which help is needed and the
source of its alleviation can be expected to lie within that
interaction. Thus it might be supposed that a psycho-
social approach in social work would be ideally suited to
the needs of the adolescent in trouble.
  Adolescence constitutes perhaps the most intensive period
of adjustment between the individual and his social environ-

ment. The intensity of this period of adjustment is
caused by the nature of the metamorphic stage between
childhood and adulthood. Here, development is not slow
and almost imperceptible as it is between middle and old
age, but sudden and startlingly obvious in the fundamental
physical changes undergone in the space of half a decade.
The corresponding emotional development involved in moving
from child to adult may take rather longer, but the transfor-
mation as a whole covers a relatively small part of the total
human life-span. In moving from complete dependence on
his family to adult independence, or from parent-determina-
tion to self-determination, the adolescent becomes involved
in crucial exploration and reconnaissance outside the home,
with friends and peers becoming at this time perhaps the
most significant others in his life. Although adolescence
may more commonly be thought of as a time of adjustment of
the adolescent to his social environment, the process is
essentially an interactionary one, in which not only the
adolescent himself but also all those who constitute his
social environment have to accommodate to a changing situation. Thus the family may go through a period of upheaval
as it adjusts to the changing roles of its adolescent members.
Schools have to come to terms with the fact that they are
not solely child-centred institutions but need to be adoles-
cent-orientated as well. The community generally acknowledges a duty to provide resources outside the home for
adolescents to engage in peer group activities, although its
provision may not always be considered adequate or appropriate for all.
    Although most societies recognize the significance of the
adolescent stage of change, the normative variations within
them are often not acknowledged or accepted. Attitudes
and behaviours vary between sub-cultures and social
classes at all life stages, but such complexity may not be
reflected in the responses of a community in its interaction
with adolescence (see Chapter seven). Standard provision
such as youth clubs may not be appropriate for some adolescent groups, while in other areas there may not be enough
of them to serve the variety necessitated by, for example,
the presence of different ethnic minority groups. Thus it
may sometimes be the case that a community's inadequate
or inappropriate responses to adolescence may be contribu-
tory factors in adolescent troubles, just as much as any
particular family difficulties or individual disorders. On
the other hand, most adolescents, like most people in other

phases of life, develop through the adolescent stage into relative harmony with themselves and their social world. A minority, however, get into trouble or difficulties and may become clients of social workers who must become involved in the interaction between adolescent and social environment, assess what is wrong and try to help. Thus adolescent-in-his-situation would seem accurately to describe the context within which both assessment and helping action should take place (Ward, 1977).

Professional social work practice, however, although claiming to focus on the interaction between the individual and his social world, has tended to overlook the latter both in the theory and in the organization of its practice. Why this should be so is discussed below. Recently, however, attempts have been made to conceptualise social work practice in models of interaction featuring all those concerned in the client's situation, including himself and the workers (Goldstein, 1973; Pincus and Minahan, 1973 and 1977). The potential contribution of such conceptual models to social work with adolescents will be explored in this chapter and questions raised about the implications for future practice.

First, however, a digression into theory and method may help to clarify how the 'social' in social work became lost for a while.

THEORY AND METHOD IN SOCIAL WORK

What is meant by the term 'theory' in social work? In an activity and profession calling itself social work it must be assumed that those in it use knowledge about human beings and their societies to make sense of problem situations presented to them and in deciding how to tackle them. Evans (1976) makes a useful distinction between explicit and implicit theory in social work. Explicit theory or 'theory of practice', he suggests, is that 'derived from the social science knowledge base of social work'. Implicit theory or 'practice theory' is that which can be inferred from the activity social workers engage in as professional practice. The distinction is not, of course, one between value-free and value-laden knowledge for propositions from the various social science disciplines are themselves culturally determined. It points, however, to the essential selectivity with which knowledge is applied in social work practice

(or, for that matter, in any other) and the values thus
assumed. Bryers (1979) has taken Evans's practice theory
formulation a step further in relation to community work,
which might be equally valid for social work, and defines it
as 'those refined, tested and clearly stated insights about
how community workers can achieve certain specified results, which have emerged from the practice of community
work'. The distinction between theory of practice and
practice theory then looks very similar to the one commonly
made, in both social work practice and training, between
social work theory and social work method.

Over the past few years, generic basic social work training courses in this country have taught casework, group
work and community work as methods of social work. A
method is defined by the Oxford English Dictionary as a
'special form of procedure'. Are casework, group work
and community work in fact methods?

Social work when it became a profession was social casework. Although its literature acknowledged the client-in-
his-situation focus, its theory of practice derived largely
from psychodynamic theories of personality development and
its practice theory looked very similar to psychotherapy.
Thus the client's theoretical 'situation' was likely to be
limited, for the purposes of social work intervention, to the
family boundary. There has been considerable debate in
recent years as to whether, in practice, social work was
ever confined to such limits. Certainly in the pre-professional social work era there had been as much concern with
the wider environment impinging on the individual, and
social work involved advocacy and political pressure to
promote or help change housing, health and education policies (Attlee, 1920). On the other hand, it has also been
suggested that in the casework of the Charity Organisation
Society the individual rather than his environment was the
focus of attention, with assessment as to the deserving or
undeserving nature of his character foremost (Woodroofe,
1962, p. 51). However, although casework constituted the
theoretical base for early professional social work, training
courses were organized on the basis of particular spheres
of work such as child care, almoning, mental health care,
etc. The casework theoretical base was borrowed from the
USA where training through the higher education system had
already begun and where a casework literature was being
established. Thus early professional social work in this
country involved the application to specialist spheres of

work of what might be termed a general casework theory, a situation which continued until the reorganization of local authority social services in 1970 and the subsequent changes to what became termed generic social work basic training.

It has been argued that social work during this time was only casework in theory and was an essentially pragmatic helping activity in practice (Davies, 1977, p. 81). Such an assertion seems to suggest that there was a theory of practice for social casework but no recognized practice theory, which is difficult to envisage. If, for example, we hold to the theory that behaviour is primarily a learning process, it seems likely that our practice theory will reflect this idea. Similarly, if we believe that people's life chances are crucially affected by their relationship to the means of production we are likely to look for ways of helping in their situation rather than in their psyches. The question then is whether social workers or the social work profession can or ought to restrict themselves to such general theories of practice, when the private ills they are expected to deal with represent an infinite number of social welfare problem permutations. The issue underlies the whole discussion about theory and practice in social work and will be re-examined later.

Returning to the question of method in social work, can casework be regarded as 'a special form of procedure'? Despite the tripartite 'methodology' provided on generic social work training courses, it is probably true to say that the majority of agency-based social workers see themselves as caseworkers, with group work and community work regarded as the specialisms of a minority (DHSS, 1978; Rees, 1978). If we look at the work carried out in social services departments, in the probation service, in hospital social work departments, in child guidance, in many voluntary social work agencies, however, we find a whole range of work done under an umbrella categorization of casework. Some of it differs in time-span of treatment (crisis intervention, long-term casework), some in relation to the roles of client and worker (task-centred casework, welfare rights advocacy) and some in respect of the number of clients or workers involved (co-counselling, family therapy), etc. These different activities could perhaps be called 'special forms of procedure', but they might be more accurately termed 'tactics', which the OED defines as 'procedure calculated to gain some end'. Thus one might argue that, as experience grows, recurring problems recognized and categorized, and skills and techniques are developed to tackle them, certain sets of tactics become adopted by the profession as appropriate 'special forms of procedure' or methods. Thus social work in most agencies staffed by 'caseworkers' probably comprises a variety of recognizable methods applied to recognizable problem situations with, in addition, the constant adaptation and application of other tactics to the as yet unclassifiable, possibly uniquely individual problems. Casework as such cannot today be regarded as a method of social work, if indeed it ever could.

Is group work a method of social work? If we accept the OED definition of method as being a procedure related to the attainment of an objective, then group work comprises a variety of methods, for different kinds of group work have different aims. Some, for example, have collective treatment aims (group therapy), others may try to incorporate both problem alleviation and prevention (mutual support groups), some have a personal development and growth function for members (therapeutic task-centred groups), others have a function of collective development or political pressure (social action or community groups). Group work can be used in treating problems, in attempting prevention or in educating people for self-help, and the only common factor is the group. There would seem to be no necessity in principle to distinguish methods of group work from other methods available to social workers. On the other hand, by lumping together into one generic term of group work a variety of methods of working in and with groups, the very real differences between them and the different approaches and skills required may be overlooked. If, as frequently happens in our experience, social work agencies assume that all groups in group work must be worker selected and directed, then group work will frequently be seen to fail. Similarly, if social workers continue to assume that group work is only for group work specialists, then what may sometimes be more relevant, more effective and more economic ways of helping will be lost to them. For example, social workers may devote much thought and time to selecting adolescents for activity-based groupwork on the basis that the peer group is a major influencing force on behaviour during adolescence. Yet the adolescents selected in this way may never meet outside the organized programme and are likely to go on being more heavily influenced by their longer-standing neighbourhood friendship groups or school cohorts with whom they spend far more time. It could well be more effective for social workers to work with existing friendship groups (as in detached youth work) or through the school (e.g. in helping to promote social education classes) (White and Brockington, 1978).

It can be argued that the practice theory of early professional casework, limited as it was to applied developmental psychology, predetermined the problems it was going to deal with as a practice. It has often been suggested in recent years that, by modelling its practice on psychotherapy, casework overlooked problems other than those of personal functioning or even reinterpreted all problems that came its way solely in such terms. Group work, on the other hand, has not suffered from criticism of problem bias, probably because it is primarily about method, in the true sense of the word. Group work comprises a number of 'special forms of procedure' which can be universally applied. Furthermore, group work methods are not exclusive to social work: they can be, and are, applied in a variety of different fields, including psychiatry, education, management and industry.

Community work, however, has also tended to have a problem bias, the polar opposite of casework. The theory of practice and practice theory of community work derive largely from political science and sociology and it has focused on the malfunctioning environment in contrast with casework's malfunctioning individual. It has assumed a social pathology rather than a personal pathology.

Community work might be described as pre-professional social work reborn or democratized. Its roots are in the earliest charity work from which, not only social work but also youth and adult education services derived. Until the 1960s community work in this country comprised chiefly those areas of voluntary welfare work which were still unprofessionalized, such as the activities promoted or supported by settlements and councils of social service. The original political pressure, social action and advocacy activity associated with early welfare work had given way, with the coming of the welfare state, to a fairly low-key coordinating role for workers in such agencies. There was no generic 'community worker' label for them any more than there was a 'social worker' one to categorize child care officers, probation officers, almoners, etc., as one professional group. However, in response to the 'rediscovery

of poverty' in the 1960s, community work became a revitali-
zed and distinct quasi-professional activity, reborn, one
might say, from a somewhat incompatible parentage of ex-
colonial British community development and US civil rights
community action. Following their American counterparts,
British social work training institutions then adopted group
work and community work as methods of social work.

But is community work a method? It is a term which can
subsume a very broad range of activities by no means all of
which would be thought of as social work by community
workers or social workers. Some of the activities might
be commonly labelled with other terms such as youth work,
race or community relations work, social planning, and
social development work. Community work is said to have
three levels of work: at 'grass roots', with neighbourhood
or community groups in promoting self-help or social
action; at inter-agency level in promoting improved service-
delivery; at policy development level as social planning
(Gulbenkian Foundation, 1968, p. 35). Where community
work has been adopted by social work agencies it has tended
to be neighbourhood work or community development, a combination of work at the first two levels. Work of this kind
involves the use of various methods and tactics, by no means
all of which have yet been clarified, categorized or refined
in the community work literature, but which include some
group work methods, advocacy, adult education methods,
political bargaining tactics, etc. Because community work
has largely developed from a belief in the relationship of
public issues to private ills in social welfare and is thus
centrally concerned about policies, its practice theory,
like that of casework, is a mirror image of its theory of
practice.

In summary, therefore, it is suggested that casework
and community work are not in themselves methods, whether
of social work or anything else. Group work is not one
single method but incorporates a number of different methods of working in and with groups to achieve various ends.

PERSONAL BELIEFS AND PROBLEM ASSESSMENT IN
SOCIAL WORK

It would seem that the curious history of social work has
brought us to a state of confusion about what we do, why we
do it and how we do it (Timms and Timms, 1977). It is

therefore important to try to distinguish between the principles of social welfare to which we adhere individually and
collectively as a profession, the assessment of particular
problems about which we expect to help, and the ways and
means – or methods of helping with those different problems.

Butrym (1976) has recently argued that the primary function of social work is the relief of suffering through various
means, both ameliorative and preventive (in which she includes influencing policy formation and change), and that
its distinctive characteristic is its relationship to actual
people, whether as individuals, families, groups or communities.   The principle, then, of help to those in difficulty
in their social situation remains clear.

Professional casework and community work are helping
activities which have been strongly linked to certain areas
of general propositional knowledge, with the result that they
have appeared to presuppose problem causation exclusively
in the person or in the social system.   Bias towards one
kind of proposition is unlikely to promote objective problem
assessment in an activity like social work where the scope
of responsibility seems at times to extend to every suffering
not dealt with by anyone else.   The contributions which
casework and community work have made to our understanding of some of the problems, and how to deal with them, are
complementary.   They do not, however, represent the only
available or relevant knowledge.   The whole gamut of
social and behavioural sciences, importantly including disciplines like philosophy, have knowledge of value for social
work.   All of it should ideally constitute social work's
'explicit theory' bank, from which it synthesizes, develops
and refines a body of knowledge and skills peculiar to its
professional task.   In so doing, one would also expect that
task itself to be refined and made more explicit so that, for
example, there would be greater clarity both inside and
outside the profession as to which kinds of suffering social
work could not relieve (a point to which we shall return).
That body of knowledge would then be social work theory –
Evans's 'implicit' or 'practice theory' according to Bryers's
definition – and would include a dynamic methodology and
tactics repertoire.

The methodological and ideological difficulties inherent
in defining the nature and causation of particular problems,
and thus possible remedies, however, remain.   By showing
that neither casework nor community work are methods in
themselves, we have not eliminated the danger of method

defining the problem. It is only too easy in social work to
become addicted to a 'special form of procedure', especially if one feels comfortable with it and finds it compatible
with one's temperament and skills. Consider, for example, the very different qualities required in advocacy
and in counselling. Then again, a worker may return from
a training course in another method stimulated and natural-
ly eager to experiment with new knowledge and skills.
There is, too, an understandable tendency in social work,
as in medicine, towards fashions in method, like the present one favouring activity groups – the popular interpretation of intermediate treatment – for children in trouble.
But the client-in-his-situation will not necessarily fit the
method of the moment and the problem variability inherent
in social work's wide remit inevitably means that it must be
a multi-methods activity, encouraged constantly to innovate.
Such argument in no way destroys the need for specialization, as we shall discuss later, any more than general medical practice does away with the need for consultants or
specialized medicine. However, it emphasizes the crucial
importance of initial assessment and helping procedures,
as in medicine, and this, in regard to young people in
trouble, was acknowledged in the 1969 Children and Young
Persons Act. Although that Act was never fully implemented, it required an initial social work assessment to be
made before any treatment decision could be made, the
social worker thus being accorded the role of the generic
practitioner (Home Office, 1970).

One might expect that the ethics of a profession such as
social work, concerned with the relief of suffering, would
dictate that neither method nor personal beliefs and ideologies should define the problem or suggest what might be
done to help. But the motivation that draws someone into
a profession of helping other people in difficulty is likely
to stem from fairly strong individual beliefs relating to the
human condition. In the case of unemployed youth, for example, one social worker may feel it important to explain
that societal values favouring market forces and profit
motives are responsible for an adolescent's unemployment,
rather than the popular media picture of the lazy young
scrounger that the young person may have come to believe
to be his mirror image. Another worker may feel it very
wrong to influence an unemployed youngster to find work
when only menial, boring jobs are available. A third
worker may see it as important to help him obtain any job,

believing that 'the devil makes work for idle hands'. Individual values are likely to determine how any professional
worker understands a situation and similarly affect how he
responds to it. Their existence will also shape the interpretation he puts on the values upheld by the profession as
a whole. For example, one worker might see the value of
client self-determination as capable of being upheld only
after putting in work on 'consciousness raising'. Another
might interpret it to such a non-directive extent that no
structure at all would be offered to the client/s within which
to respond. On the other hand, given what we know about
the social construction of reality, complete objectivity is
hardly a realistic goal for social workers to strive after
(Berger and Luckmann, 1972). Nor, arguably, is it a
desirable one, for passion and energy arising from strong
personal beliefs can make as important a contribution to
helping as their absence can limit it. It is, too, the very
stuff of innovation.

Professional values, important though they may be as
guiding principles, do not in themselves ensure against differential interpretation in assessing and deciding on the
social work task. On the other hand, it is inconceivable
that, for example, in a social services department generic
team the caseload of a social worker disciple of Freud
could all be problems of personal dysfunctioning while those
of his Marxist colleague are all traceable to political disadvantage. Similarly, advocacy with the Department of
Health and Social Security may be the appropriate helping
response in the case of the truanting child whose mother
cannot afford to buy him shoes. But no form of advocacy
is likely to succeed in getting his class mate back to school,
who is distressed by parental disputes and conflict and
afraid of what might happen if he is away from home all day
long. And neither the family counselling that might help
there, nor welfare rights advocacy, is likely to end the
truanting of a group of boys in the last year at school who
are bored with the conventional curriculum.

Each social worker is faced with a prime, professional
responsibility for continuous self-assessment, for awareness of his personal beliefs, ideologies, prejudices and
predilections and of where they may help and where hinder.
But he also needs some conceptual tools to help guard
against the natural tendency to simplify problem definition
and methods of helping in an area of concern as wide as
that covered by social work.

A few social work theorists in the USA in recent years
have been trying to develop such conceptual tools, endeav-
ouring to avoid the separate emphasis on the client or his
situation that traditional casework and community work
practice seem to have produced.   Theorists such as Goldstein (1973), Pincus and Minahan (1973 and 1977) and Middleman and Goldberg (1974) have tried to devise models
which are capable of allowing a wide view of the client in
interaction with his environment, for many different kinds
of intervening factors in the situation, and for a variety of
types and methods of social work intervention, calling for
different professional roles and relationships for the
worker in carrying out his helping task.

A DYNAMIC CONCEPTUALIZATION OF SOCIAL WORK

To view the client in interaction with his situation is to
view a moving picture, a dynamic relationship such as we
described for the normal adolescent and his social environment (see also Chapter two).   Implicit in such a view is
reciprocity, process and a complex web of cause and
effect.   In addition, it is a process of interaction in which
the social worker enters as a significant actor himself who,
by design or otherwise, will change it some extent.   So the
social worker must view a moving picture with himself as
part of that picture.   Many other actors and factors also
play parts either directly or indirectly, and to greater or
less effect,   so that a dynamic conceptualization of the
client-in-his-situation has to be more than merely two-
dimensional.   It needs to be a multi-dimensional moving
model, capable of revealing the different intensities of involvement which will make it possible to distinguish critical paths for intervention, for the variables in the situation
- be they people, policies or institutions - will also be dif-
ferentially open to influence from social work intervention.
As the social work proceeds, the model must also be able
to help the worker constantly to reassess and evaluate, so
that new or different problems can be identified, critical
paths for intervention illuminated, and different methods of
work adopted for the different kinds of intervention judged
to be appropriate.

The concept of a system

A basis for building dynamic models of social work of that
kind has been borrowed from general system theory, a
theory which Davies has described as a 'general science of
wholeness, valid for all systems whatever the nature of
their component parts - electrons, cells, ants, men as individuals or in groups - and whatever the nature of the relations between them' (Davies, 1977, p. 89). As Davies explains, the use of system concepts in social work has been
adapted from the work of the biologist Von Bertalaffny, who
sought to find a means of conceptualizing living, spontaneous and complex beings in non-mechanistic terms, but in
ways which recognized their patterns of growth and organization. The term system used in this way may describe
each of the component parts of a social work problem situation, as indeed of any other human or social situation, and
immediately links the client and his situation into their
interaction. We see the client as a system within a situation comprising many other interacting systems such as
family members, peer groups, school, etc. A system may
be defined as being composed of elements related in a stable
but active, causal network. One can then distinguish in
the social work situation three kinds of systems: intra-
personal systems which are individual persons, inter-personal systems of which most people belong to a large variety, such as the family, friendship groups, work groups,
etc., and socio-cultural or socio-economic systems which
comprise organizations, churches and other institutions,
bureaucracies, communities etc.
  It may be thought that the caring has gone out of social
work if we depersonalize the client by referring to him in
the same terms as a 'thing' like an organization. By so
doing, however, we do not need to lose sight of the human-
ity of our client, for the notion of his 'active causal network' is not only consistent with many religious beliefs and
principles from philosophy, but also with the body of knowledge from psychology on personality development, so central to the original casework method. The very notion of
mental or personality 'disturbance' is indicative of just such
a network in each of us.
  On the other hand, it can be argued that systems are in
fact all human, that inter-personal and social systems are
composed of people and that the concept of 'it' to understand an organization or an agency, for example, is

decidedly unhelpful in an activity such as social work. It
is easy to drift into the assumption that 'it' is a fixed,
static factor. However, as systems, the Social Services
Department, the DHSS, the School and so on are actually
people, related in active, causal networks and, as such,
in principle as amenable to our efforts to influence as are
our clients.

The notion of 'functioning', which in traditional casework
related to the ability of the individual client to fit comfort-
ably into his situation, may then be usefully extended to,
say, service delivery systems where they form part of the
social environment of actual or potential social work
clients. Dysfunctions in such systems where, for example,
they have been especially created to support family and individual systems, may actually contribute more to social
work problems than their service delivery assuages.
Thus, for example, two of the polar concerns of traditional
casework and community work – individual functioning and
service delivery functioning – can be brought into a single
conceptual framework from the outset, and their relative
merits in any particular case considered. Similarly, two
bodies of substantive knowledge – about the individual and
about society – are conceptually linked, in the first instance
for attempting to understand and assess problems and then,
to consider the range of possible courses for action. It
provides us at least with a basic conceptual structure within which, whether we are at heart psychologists or socio-
logists, we can be helped to integrate and use knowledge
from different disciplines as appropriate.

The idea of a system comprising elements related in a
stable but active causal network serves also to remind us
that a personality or social system is something besides the
sum of its parts: it has discrete properties which can be
recognized. A particular network will have a meaning and
a function for its individual members, although they may by
no means be the same for each of them. An example in
social work with adolescents might be the family, whereby
everyone involved in the situation would agree that it existed as a system but its meaning and function might well be
very different for the parents, the younger siblings and the
adolescent, and could have very different interpretations
put on it by, say, the schoolmaster, the police or the psychiatrist.

Similarly, we are reminded that change in one part of a
system is likely to have some effect on its other parts. In

traditional casework that assumption underlay its psychodynamic intervention. Do we, however, always remember
it when working for change in other kinds of systems?
Perhaps in social work with families we are sensitive to
such a possibility, but how often in social work agencies is
it used as a positive tactic to achieve a policy change in the
interests of clients, as might be the case in community
work?

The assertion of stability in a system need not imply that
a system is in a constant state of harmonious balance and
that there is never internal conflict or disruption. The
social systems 'functionalist' school of sociology has been
criticized for assuming a consensus, co-operative model of
society, but in using a systems framework for conceptualizing social work practice situations no such implication is
being made. As Evans (1976, p. 189) points out, we are
here referring essentially to causal interdependence.
Conflict, on the contrary, can often develop within systems
and often changes them in the process. The arrival, for
example, of a new head to a school may be the cause of an
outbreak of conflict within the system precisely because of
intent to change the system, but the school remains a recognizable school system. Even personality systems suffer
from internal disruption, as the existence of the profession
of psychiatry might suggest, although they rarely collapse
totally. Similarly, social systems such as the family may
frequently suffer internal disruption and change shape, as
well as function and meaning, for its members. Obviously,
too, they may also cease to exist altogether as, for example, when a family dies out or an organization is disbanded.
Thus the notion of stability does not deny conflict or change
in systems, but suggests what has been described as a
'steady state' in which systems develop and change, but
nevertheless maintain a recognizable existence (Goldstein,
1973, p. 116).

It will be clear from the above that systems are composed
of sub-systems and may themselves be sub-systems of
numerous other systems. Such conceptualization rather
neatly portrays the complexity of the individual. For one
person is, for example, a member of a family, of a peer
group, of an extended family network, of different friendship groups, status groups, work groups, professional
groups, etc. Any social situation, therefore, is likely to
contain patterns of complex and diverse loyalties between
and within sub-systems and systems which may considerably

influence a social worker's ability to help effectively, but which may not always be self-evident.

Implicit in the discussion so far, which shows how the concept of a system has the capability to provide the necessary dynamic quality required for theoretical models in social work, is the open nature of systems. Nature itself is a picture of interacting open biological systems and, similarly, social systems are constantly engaged in exchange with, and influence by, other social systems in the environment. Davies (1977, p. 107) has illustrated in a helpful way how the idea of systems importing energy from each other, transforming it and exporting it in a converted form as inputs for other systems, can aid understanding of the complex interactions in many social work situations, where the energy exchange may not necessarily be positive for the systems involved. For example, Jordan (1972) has pointed out the dangers in social work with centrifugal families of taking the deviant-labelled child into care. First, it may only serve to confirm that label and, second, it is likely to reinforce the dysfunctional family dynamics and possibly contribute to another scapegoating and rejection. Third, the social worker can become drawn into the family dynamics as a collusive force, confirming rather than challenging its dysfunctional features. In such a case there is negative energy exchange, in that the energy introduced into the family system by the social worker in the interests of the rejected child is transformed and used by the family against him instead. Although some of the rather technical discussion in the literature (e.g. Hearn, 1969; Janchill, 1969) on the properties of open systems may, it is feared, often block rather than stimulate the imagination of social workers (a case of negative energy exchange?), the idea that the behaviour of people is understandable chiefly in relation to their interaction with each other is, surely, fundamental to social work.

The multiplicity and variability of exchanges between open systems can serve to remind us that there may be any number of points or levels of interaction at which the 'helping' intervention of social work could, in principle, be aimed to bring about the desired change. All of those ways may not be appropriate in every case, but the broader view may suggest new approaches and at least may induce us to explain, if only to ourselves, why some of them may not be useful ways of proceeding. Implicit in this idea, too, is the fact that problems experienced at one system level, such as the

individual, do not necessarily have to be dealt with solely
at that level, for change in one system, for example in a
youth club, may improve the situation for not just one particular adolescent but for all the members.

Related to the notion of open systems is that of system
boundaries which must, by definition, exist but which are
obviously permeable. However, permeability is a relative
idea and can be useful both in understanding social work
problems and weighing up the alternatives for action. Consider, for example, the problem of the child born of an ex-
ceptionally self-contained and engrossed couple, who can
never feel part of the family system because the family unit
does not exist – the couple has, in fact, remained a dyad;
or the reverse, the child whose own system boundaries are
constantly violated by suffocating parents (see Laing, 1960;
Laing and Esterson, 1964). In deciding how to help one is
likely to take into account the relative ease or difficulty in
working across system boundaries and to choose to work
where they are more permeable, more adaptable and open
to change. Thus, in the case of an adolescent diagnosed
as schizophrenic, the social worker may choose to start to
work with the adolescent himself, with the parents, or with
the family as a system, depending on which system he perceives to be most amenable to change.

A combination of systems properties has appeal in understanding what we are trying to do in social work. It emphasizes both their dynamic nature, their state of constant
movement and adjustment, and their essential wholeness,
for each system is more than a collection of sub-systems
and has a meaning and an integrity of its own. The steady-
state nature of systems reminds us that, although we speak
of systems constantly changing, and in social work we are
aiming to achieve some kind of change for good, the change
is likely to be slow and not necessarily very dramatic.
Perhaps we should speak not of change, but of adaptation
which gives a truer impression of the scale of time often
needed for any real change to take effect. The idea of the
social worker as a change-agent does seem to overstate and
perhaps distort the nature of helping in social work (Lippitt,
Watson and Westley, 1958, p. 11). The dynamic nature of
systems can also be useful in reminding us that there is
always a history to the present situation, the development
of which is likely to be crucial in understanding the problem
of the moment and, particularly, in assessing the possibilities for future change or adaptation. In traditional social

work the social history of the client has long been regarded
as important for the purpose of assessment, but the principle is equally valid for understanding any system and deciding how to intervene in it, be it group, organization or community.

Using a systems framework

The interaction of different systems as the focus of social
work intervention is implicit in several of the models of
social work practice which have been offered in recent
years. In those of Goldstein (1973) and Pincus and Minahan (1973 and 1977) quite explicit use of systems concepts
is made which offers different but highly complementary
help to the social worker, particularly in the early assessment and intervention stages of social work. As already
indicated, the activity or craft of social work is itself a
dynamic process in which assessment, intervention and
evaluation are, and must be, continuous and cyclic, for the
worker's involvement will of itself alter the situation
(whether as intended or otherwise) and thus require constant reappraisal. In this way, any benefit that conceptual models may offer in the assessment and initial helping
stages is likely to reflect throughout the cycle.
   Goldstein (1973) uses analysis of system properties to
provide an initial theoretical famework for understanding a
situation as presented to the social worker.* Using a
hypothetical case, he identifies and describes the various
systems interacting in it and affecting it, systems ranging
from the individual client, Bill, an adolescent referred because of a drug offence, to siblings, parents, peer group,
probation service, community service centre, court,
school, neighbourhood, local industry and local community.
A fairly simple diagram, as he shows, can illustrate the
interaction of large and small systems, or of a hierarchy of
sub-systems within a major system, and how they are affect-

* There will be no attempt here to portray the entire social
work practice model of either Goldstein or the other theorists discussed. The intention is to focus attention on those
elements considered to be of particular relevance to a truly
psycho-social approach to the client-in-his-situation.
Thus the portion of Goldstein's model discussed above represents but one part of it.

ing one another. It is capable of revealing 'the complex
nature of the larger social problem as well as its impact on
specific persons or groups'. Similarly, the exercise of
identification and description of what is known about all the
systems involved can help 'identify the points ... where the
most effective intervention is possible' (Goldstein, 1973,
p. 110).

The implication throughout Goldstein's primarily American model for practice is that social work is organized and
operated on an individual referrals basis, an assumption
which holds equally well for social work services in this
country. Certain problems arise here which will be examined later. However, such problems apart, Goldstein
offers in his systems framework not only a means of examining the client in interaction with his social environment,
involving a considerable variety of potentially relevant information about client and environment, but also a tactic for
holding on to several distinct but interlocking bodies of information while trying to identify and assess possible courses of action. That tactic involves a simple skill, rarely
seen in social work agencies to our knowledge, but one
which is more generally adopted in community work, namely
the use of diagrammatic presentation for understanding complex situations. Great importance seems to be attached in
social work agencies to the need for records for such purposes (as well as for other purposes of course). However, records in social work are often verbose and confusing and it is to be hoped that where the sole aim of recording is to illuminate worker and agency understanding of particular practice situations, diagrammatic techniques and
methods will become more widely practised as they have
been by other professions, such as management, also concerned with human relations.

Goldstein is helpful, then, in providing a first frame of
reference for understanding the complexity of a referred
problem. With it one can describe and plot all the systems
involved and the nature and significance of the interaction
between them, on the basis of which decisions about goals
and methods can be made with a broader and clearer view.
Thus Goldstein, as it were, sets the scene. Pincus and
Minahan (1973 and 1977) classify the actors and identify the
principal roles. Their model offers specific role categor-
izations for understanding who needs our help and who we
must try and influence in order to be effective in that help.
'The key element of our model is a classification of the types

of systems in relation to which the social worker carries
out his role' (Pincus and Minahan, 1977, p. 81).   In effect
they are trying to prod the worker to ask the right kinds of
questions at the outset about the particular situation, and to
assist him to make decisions appropriate primarily to it
rather than to agency or worker ideology or methodology.
   Thus, their first question seems to be 'Who am I, as a
social worker?'   The social worker is a change-agent and
is, of course, a system though he is not classified as such.
However, he is employed by the social work agency which is
the change-agent system, to which he thus bears some
ccountability.   Pincus and Minahan identify the client
system as the person, family, group, organization or community which in fact 'engages the services of the worker ...
and is the expected beneficiary of the worker's efforts'
(Pincus and Minahan, 1977, p. 81).   In other words, the
client system comprises whoever is the willing recipient of
the worker's services.   Thus Pincus and Minahan rather
neatly remind us of the inherent dilemma for the semi-pro-
fessional helper, the dilemma between accountability to
those who employ him and to those he is employed to serve
professionally.   Behind that dilemma are often unspoken
questions about who sanctions the work and whether those
who sanction it can then have the right to override professional decisions about particular cases or, indeed, should
influence the nature of the work in any way.   In social work
in this country one can isolate four possible different sectors of interest here: first, the society, or the community
in general, which sanctions a general professional activity
such as social work and legislates to require a few specific
activities to be carried out in certain situations;   second,
the different agencies or authorities which actually employ
social workers, many of which are required by law to carry
out general and specific social work activities;   third, the
consumers of social work services;   fourth, social workers
themselves, individually and collectively.   In the case of
supervision orders, for instance, it is Parliament which
passes the legislation, the government which enables it to
be enacted, the magistrates who sanction the use of compulsory supervision in specific cases, and the social work
agency which provides the resources to enable it to be
carried out.   In addition, the elected councillors, the
agency's professional managers, the social workers and, by
virtue of the reciprocal nature of supervision, the consumers themselves, may all have some say over how it should

be implemented. The conflicting values and clashes of
interest between all these parties may be one reason for the
reduction in supervision orders now being made by courts.

In their model, Pincus and Minahan acknowledge the possible clashes of interest between those involved, directly
or indirectly, in carrying out a piece of social work. In
particular, they point to the possibility that the social work
agency itself may need to adapt or change in order to provide a more effective service, although they concede that
'the worker will be operating with different sanctions, constraints and opportunities when his own agency, as contras-
ted to an outside system, becomes a target for change'
(Pincus and Minahan, 1977, p. 81). Such a statement
carries a host of implications for all the parties involved in
social work which have hardly begun to be faced.

Pincus and Minahan also acknowledge that the consumers
of social work services may sometimes be unwilling ones
who have not engaged the services of the worker. An adolescent referred for social work because he has offended
might be an example. Thus the term 'client system' implies
an unwritten form of contract between worker and prospec-
tive consumer of his services, or a sanction from the client,
for Pincus and Minahan distinguish the existence or the need
in social work for two kinds of sanction to underwrite a
contract: a general sanction deriving from professional and
public recognition of competence, and a specific sanction
from the consumer to receive the particular service.
Where that specific sanction is not given by the consumer,
but derives from the community or society, the worker has
no client system. The client is then the 'target system',
'which refers to those people the change agent needs to influence in order to accomplish the goals of his change
effort' (Pincus and Minahan, 1977, p. 82).

Thus Pincus and Minahan's model acknowledges the reciprocal nature of social work helping which requires the co-
operation of the recipient in order to be effective. Social
work helping of all kinds may then usefully be distinguished
from the medical model of 'treatment' with its connotations
of 'doing to' and passive reception of drugs or surgery. It
is perhaps unfortunate that traditional casework literature
has been characterized by the concept of treatment, despite
the lip-service paid to client self-determination and the implication of a shared social work activity.

A target system, then, in Pincus and Minahan's model
constitutes any system the worker needs to influence in

order to achieve the goals jointly agreed between the worker
and client system. A target system may thus be an unwilling client, as already indicated, where the worker must
first gain the reluctant consumer's acknowledgment of the
validity of social work intervention and confidence in its
worth. It may also be a willing client system as, for example, when worker and client have agreed on a goal concerned with improving personal functioning. Often it may
not be the client system at all, but one or several systems
in the client's situation which may crucially affect the
chances of achieving the goals set. Sometimes it might be
the social work agency itself, particularly where, for example, the worker comes to feel that a particular policy has
begun to operate against the purpose it was designed to
serve. A recent example of such dysfunctioning might be
the structure of residential care for young offenders, which
has been thought by many social workers to be a hindrance
rather than a help (Tutt, 1974). In practice, of course,
there will be different targets for different goals at different times during any particular social work process.
   Similarly, there will be different 'action systems' employed (Pincus and Minahan, 1977, p. 83). Such systems
are those with the potential and willingness to assist the
worker and client in their tasks. Thus Pincus and Minahan
acknowledge that social workers do not and should not work
in isolation, that successful social work also requires numerous inputs from other sources in the situation like family,
friends, institutions and agencies, professional groups,
community groups and so on. They also thereby remind us
of the need to maximize helping resources, and to try to
create and develop them as well, through support and encouragement to voluntary groups and volunteers, for example. We are further reminded that social work is not just
a question of direct helping from one worker to one client.
There can be various ways of helping through indirect
means, such as through other people.
   In summary, then, a combination of ideas developed from
general system theory can provide a dynamic conceptual
framework to aid us in trying to see the whole picture of the
client-in-his-situation. We can thereby identify and describe all those involved, analyse the nature of their interaction, and, from such a wider view and analysis, better
determine goals appropriate to that particular situation and
how best to achieve them. An example of how such a framework might be used to examine and understand a case involv-

ing adolescents is given by Jones (1976). Its use need not
be restricted to initial assessment but, as pointed out earlier, can serve throughout the cycle of social work as a
means of evaluating any change resulting from social work
intervention, for modifying goals, planning new phases of
work, etc.

COMMON ASSUMPTIONS OF UNITARY MODELS

The wider view of a problem situation afforded by the use of
a systems framework is also likely to promote the choice of
more appropriate ways of helping, since alternative courses
for action should thereby become more evident. However,
the framework is not primarily concerned with means or
method. Some misunderstanding and confusion may have
arisen on this point, for the models of social work practice,
such as those of Goldstein and Pincus and Minahan, have
come to be known as a 'unitary approach' to social work
practice or 'integrated social work methods' (e.g. Hunter
and Ainsworth, 1975; Specht and Vickery, 1977). One can
see why this has happened, given the curious development of
a tripartite so-called 'methodology' already discussed, and
the unitary authors themselves seem to have started from the
assumption that the activities hitherto comprised in casework, in social work with groups, and in community work,
together constitute social work practice. On that basis
they each attempt to elaborate and synthesize the elements
common to these activities and to arrive at a fully comprehensive conceptual model of social work practice. Goldstein (1973) for example, uses a third of his book to provide, within what he calls a process model of strategies for,
targets of, and phases in, social work practice, what
amounts to a checklist for all social work situations. In a
similar vein, Pincus and Minahan (1973) devote half their
book to a detailed analysis of the activities involved in the
eight practice skill areas which they believe encompass and
constitute the process of all social work practice. Middleman and Goldberg (1974), similarly, detect six skill areas
which incorporate twenty-seven different 'behaviours' for
social workers, and use a large part of their book to illustrate the application of these behaviours in different social
work situations. One questions whether it is either realistic or helpful to students or practitioners to attempt such
detailed and comprehensive models of a practice which is

still in the throes of development and having to adjust, in
this country at least, to the considerable structural changes
of recent years. Is clarity and rigour of thought about
what, why and how we do social work, which has become so
important in the light of the enormous scope and range of
generic practice, best promoted by conceptual manuals
which these models are in danger of becoming? The trouble
with manuals is that they often belie their comprehensive
appearance; one is left with a nagging suspicion that there
might even be nine practice skill areas or even thirty-four
behaviours! It may be more helpful at this early stage of
generic conceptualisation in social work, to think in terms
of several simple conceptual frameworks, common to all
social work but relative to different phases or aspects of
practice, in the way that the systems framework already
discussed relates primarily to assessment. These could
then be applied to specialist areas or foci of practice, such
as work with adolescents, to draw together and refine in
greater depth a range of relevant knowledge, skills and
methods of helping.

The ingredients of social work

One very simple framework for understanding the basic ingredients in the doing of social work can be devised from
three elements found in the unitary models already cited,
and it might help students to sort out their own responses to
what still seems to be the problematical question of 'What do
we do when we do social work?' (Timms and Timms, 1977,
p. 9). The framework would show the self as the tool used
in the doing of social work, relationships as the medium
through which it is carried out, and social learning as the
helping product of effective social work.
    The importance of the person of the social worker is par-
ticularly emphasized by Goldstein. It would probably be
generally agreed that a social worker brings acquired knowledge, learned skills and shared professional values to his
job, and that his practice is a product of the fusion of these
factors with his own personality. Goldstein suggests that
the 'style' of the worker is the central mechanism affecting
the quality of social work provided, one which transcends
technical knowledge and skill, vital though these are. He
sees style as a composite of personal and technical characteristics, with the personal characteristics being the more

determinate (Goldstein, 1973).   Social worker, know thyself...! Goldstein cites research in the USA to support
his view, and in this country the fairly limited amount of
consumer research in social work would also tend to confirm
the significance of the worker's personal characteristics to
clients of social work (e.g. Mayer and Timms, 1970; Sainsbury, 1975; Rees, 1978).   The implications of this fact for
more effective social work have not perhaps been sufficiently explored.   How often are social workers ready to accept
that their own style may be more helpful for some kinds of
people and situations than for others and, for example, to
suggest transfer of cases?   In the case of adolescents,
there is certainly evidence which confirms the significance
of social worker style, sometimes combined with preference
for one form of intervention over another (Anon., 1975).
Adolescents in trouble, in particular, often state a preference for activity-based group work programmes and, within
these, differentiate between the styles of the individual
social workers (Jones, 1979).   Adolescents in care also
show a preference for differing regimes and styles of worker
contact (Page and Clark, 1977; Walter, 1978).
   The use of the relationship with a client to influence and
help him has long been a central feature of social casework
literature.   The unitary authors, however, emphasize the
significance for effective social work of relationships not
only with the client but also with significant others in the
situation.   Pincus and Minahan (1977, p. 84) believe that
the preoccupation in social work with relationships with
clients has led to a tendency to view professional relationships as essentially collaborative.   If, however, one considers all of the systems in Pincus and Minahan's model
with whom the worker must have effective relationships in
order himself to be effective, i.e. change-agent system,
target systems and action systems as well as the client
system, then the significance of different kinds of relating
becomes apparent.   For it is clear that, in order most
effectively to serve the interests of clients in a situation
requiring advocacy, for example, collaboration with the
authority concerned may well not prove successful.   For
example, a particularly problematic issue for social workers with adolescents in trouble concerns the initial police
inquiry on a juvenile they may wish to prosecute.   How
much information can or should be given to the police by the
social worker and how should it be presented?   If a worker
feels that prosecution is likely to cause more harm than

good, he may want to withhold information which he considers to be confidential or which he fears may paint too negative a picture of the adolescent.   The cost of doing so,
however, may well be less trust and less consultation in the
future between social workers and the police and thereby
possibly be of less benefit to the adolescents who get into
trouble.   On the other hand, in order to achieve the necessary collaboration with one's client, particularly, say, with
an adolescent in trouble, a prior relationship which is
essentially one of bargaining has often to be entered into.
Thus Pincus and Minahan (1977, pp. 84-6) isolate three
broad categories of professional relationships in social
work: collaborative, bargaining and conflictual.   Goldstein (1973, pp. 9-11) sees professional relationships as
'affiliative interaction', an idea which, when applied to relationships with other systems, can be as significant as for
those with clients.   For example, relationships with other
agencies, other professionals etc., are likely to be dynamic
and therefore to affect the service one can offer to future
clients, as well as present ones.   Similarly, we are reminded of the importance of forging and building relationships, within and outside our own agencies, in anticipation
of likely clients, i.e. as a preventive measure.   Examples
in work with adolescents might be the building of sound relationships with local school teachers, youth workers,
policemen etc. (see Chapter four).
    Social learning, as the helping product of effective social
work, ties in with the broadly educative goals of much community work and moves social work away from the medical
treatment model.   Goldstein proposes the concept of social
learning and argues that, in so far as social work objectives are invariably concerned with adjustment and change -
and not only on the part of clients - adjustment and change
can only derive from a logical series of learning experiences, irrespective of the methods or techniques employed to
achieve it.   The process of social learning is one which
we are all going through throughout our lives, but Goldstein
points out that it is relatively casual and uneven apart from
critical developmental periods such as adolescence.   He
distinguishes social learning in social work from the casual
nature of other social learning by the intensity of the need
to be fulfilled or the goal to be achieved.   Learning, as
crisis intervention assumes, is more effective at critical
moments and, almost by definition, social work can be said
to be concerned with critical events.   So he sees social

learning related to goal attainment within a managed process of problem solving. Thus the notion of social learning suggests that the worker has to try to develop 'those conditions most conducive to learning ... the primary objective of practice is providing that context' (Goldstein, 1973, p. 8).

The skill of enabling, fundamental to community work, is also concerned with trying to promote conditions in which people can best develop their own capacities to deal with problems. But promoting an environment most conducive to learning can make very different demands upon social workers and social work agencies from those that a treatment model imposes. For example, the concept of social learning itself implies that people learn from interaction with each other and suggests, perhaps, a greater use of groups in social work methods than the present referrals system of most social work agencies tends to allow. It might also suggest a greater exploitation of the social work team as a group, for tackling problems both inside and outside the agency, than is presently the case in so many agencies where the team is more a collection of individual systems than a system itself. The recent report of Stevenson and Parsloe makes just this point in asking whether the meaning of the word team in social work is closer to that of a football team or of a tennis team: 'Our studies suggest that teams vary greatly along a continuum from football to tennis, but that, in general, the analogy with tennis teams is nearer to the reality of social work in the area teams' (DHSS, 1978, p. 307). Furthermore, the enabler as worker has a far less obvious authority than the doctor in the treatment model. His role is more akin to that of the youth worker who, rather than having authority ascribed to him, has to create it very largely by the force of his own personality. Perhaps too, a greater degree of flexibility is demanded, not only in worker/client relationships but also in methods of work and in the use of 'action systems' other than professionals. Some move in this direction has been made, for example in work with offenders through such projects as New Careers, whereby ex-offenders are employed as social workers; or in projects which offer workshops on social skills for adolescents. Generally speaking, however, such initiatives in social learning remain with special projects and are rarely found as part of the repertoire of the main social work agencies of their workers.

The scope of social work activity

Another fairly simple conceptual framework with which to
describe the scope of social work activity is provided by
Middleman and Goldberg (1973).   Their quadrant (Figure
3.1) is based on assumptions which are shared by all the
unitary authors and indicates four major areas of social
work activity:

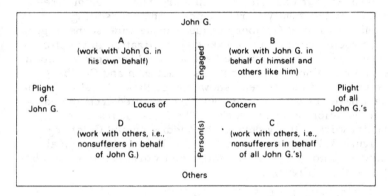

FIGURE 3.1   (reproduced from Middleman and Goldberg,
1973, p. 19)

Sector A represents work with a particular client, family
or group, etc. on a problem which is specific to him/them
and thus primarily for his/their benefit.   Sector B represents work with a particular client, family or group, etc.
on a problem which is theirs but which is also shared by
other people who may not necessarily have been referred.
A worker might, for example, help the working single
parent of one latchkey child to seek facilities through the
local school or church for immediate after-school care not
only of her child but of others in the locality in a similar
situation.   Or one might work with a small group of parents
to create a holiday play scheme for the children of a whole
neighbourhood or estate.   Sector C work is chiefly concerned with categories of suffering or specific problem
areas and how to alleviate them.   It does not centre on a
particular client.   Such activity might be classified as preventive work and could include research on social problems
recurrent in social work (e.g. through regular analysis of
referrals), efforts to improve social work management and

service delivery, and measures designed to influence social
policy and planning. For example, analysis of neighbourhood delinquency rates throughout a city can provide a guide
as to how resources can best be allocated and distributed.
Sector D work is again based on the problems of particular
persons but requires the mobilization of external 'action
systems' to help on behalf of the particular sufferers.
Work of this nature could include all kinds of advocacy and
measures, for example, to help a pregnant schoolgirl rejected by her family to receive care and counselling.

Middleman and Goldberg argue that the wide scope of generic social work activity makes specialization in practice
inevitable. Indeed, there have always been specialization
divisions in social work but, as Middleman and Goldberg
point out and as has been shown here, those divisions in the
past have not been planned but have resulted from the natural evolution of social work. The four-quadrant model of
social work activity devised by Middleman and Goldberg
(Figure 3.1) expresses what they believe to be a logical
division into two main specialisms of work, with overlap between them (Figure 3.2).

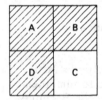 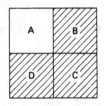

Social service delivery   Social policy-planning

FIGURE 3.2 (reproduced from Middleman and Goldberg,
1973, p. 29)

Thus, one (ABD), social service delivery, or what might
in this country be called referrals-based work, follows
'the demands of the client task', whilst the other (CBD),
social policy-planning, is based on 'the demands of the
social task' and starts from a more general or macro-level
of social welfare. If we apply that model to social work
in present-day social services departments, it seems likely
that we would find the bulk of the work to be closer to the
referrals-based area of activity than to the other. Where
work centred on Middleman and Goldberg's sector C does
occur, such as for example with specializations based on
particular need areas or client groups such as the men-

tally handicapped or ethnic minorities etc., the specialist
workers are either situated at a higher level than the area
team or, if at area level, they operate exclusively on a referrals basis by receiving all referrals in that particular
category (DHSS, 1978). Perhaps in the field of social
work with adolescents some patterns of work are appearing
similar to Middleman and Goldberg's model, possibly as a
result of the recent interest in, and availability of grant aid
for, intermediate treatment projects. However, these too
often derive only from referrals, in that the young people
enabled to join in such activities are drawn from existing
caseloads, and do not start from the demands of the social
task as Middleman and Goldberg's model would require.
Thus in, say, area team work with adolescents of a truly
social policy-planning nature, the specialists would start
from an examination of the needs of the area and of the
client grouping as a whole, with their priorities being
determined primarily from such an overview (see Jones and
Kerslake, 1979). Out of it, work with, or on behalf of,
specific groups (sectors B and D) could develop, but such
groups would not necessarily relate to the caseload referral
pattern.

The field of social work

A final conceptual framework which expresses the common
assumptions of the unitary authors is provided by Carol
Meyer (1976) who analyses the field of social work in terms
of context, contours and content. Social work, she
argues, is a service which, given the particular socio-
economic nature of western and European life today, has to
be viewed within a context of normality or universality of
need. Public services of all kinds which are now commonly
accepted have tended to develop out of a need continuum
ranging from relative abnormality, or the needs of the few,
to relative normality or the needs of the majority, or from a
view of individual pathology to one of social pathology. An
example common in the community work experience of the
author is the case of the pedestrian crossing. Local residents will press for one, warning the authorities of the
traffic dangers for children and old people at that particular spot, but all too often their views are disregarded until
after several accidents have proved their point. Thus,
after a period of treating the matter as a question of indi-

vidual pathology ('those people constantly going on about
that road ... trouble-makers') the authorities will then
accept that a social problem exists which requires a community decision, i.e. a social policy.

Meyer points out that the contours of social work are, of
course, defined by social policy. However, given the
nature of social policy development out of the individual-
social pathology continuum, she argues that social workers
have a key role to play in feeding back information and recommendations on the changing social welfare needs and conditions at consumer or grassroots level, in order properly
to influence relevant social policy. Thus the field of
social work includes a legitimate policy-shaping function, a
point emphasized by all the unitary authors. But Meyer
suggests that, whereas in its early years social work had a
strong policy-making and campaigning function, in recent
years professional social work has largely abandoned that
function, expecting now to be informed by policy rather than
to form it (Meyer, 1976, pp. 93-105). However, it is the
case that social workers have begun to use their professional associations to some extent for policy-shaping purposes as, for example, when the British Association of
Social Workers campaigned for the implementation of the
proposals of the Finer Report (1974) on services for single
parent families, against the ideology underlying some sections of the Children Act 1975, and for the further implementation of the Children and Young Persons Act 1969.

The third side of Meyer's triangle is the knowledge content of social work which, in common with the other unitary
authors, she believes must necessarily derive from a
number of different disciplines in the humanities, social and
behavioural sciences in order that the dual functions of
social work, that of immediate help with individual problems
and the longer-term help of a more preventive nature
achieved through involvement in policy-shaping, may be
effectively carried out:

The social work practitioner will need to be expert in his
comprehension of the nature of human beings living in a
complex urban environment, and his particular expertise
will be found in his knowledge of how the person and the
situation reinforce each other or, more likely, fail to do
so. In our view of the unit of attention being the individual in his life style we have left behind the concept of
the clinically defined disease, and we may even have put
aside the requirement of becoming a client in order to be
helped by a social worker (Meyer, 1976, pp. 162-3).

Speaking of the USA, Meyer considers that important areas
of knowledge are still omitted from social workers' education, significantly those covering major aspects of our
social world such as economics, politics, planning, government, etc. The situation is not likely to be very different
in this country. For example, the writer regularly explores with social work students the extent of their knowledge and understanding of the operations of central and
local government; of the differences between the theory and
the practice of elected member and employed officer roles;
of the nature and function of planning in local government
and its relationship to social policy; of welfare economics,
as opposed merely to welfare rights, etc. It is rare to
find more than a shred of knowledge in these areas.

SUMMARY AND CONCLUSIONS

It has been argued here that social work with adolescents,
as indeed all professional social work helping, must pro-
ceed logically from the principles of social welfare it
claims to uphold, through assessment of the problems it
seeks to tackle, to the methods it uses to do so. However,
until recently social work has been dominated by, and
brought to a state of conceptual confusion through, the
false assumption that there are three basic ways of doing
social work, i.e. casework, group work or community
work. The historical reasons for this assumption, and the
concomitant failure to distinguish social work theory from
method, have been discussed as a basis for considering the
contribution that the recent unitary conceptualizations of
social work can make towards greater clarity of thought and
action about social work principles, problems and methods
of practice. It has been suggested that the greatest potential at this stage is to be found in a variety of simple conceptual frameworks relating to different aspects of practice, rather than in the use of one or other of the complete
unitary models.
　Social work with adolescents presents a particularly
good practice example to use in examining the contribution
of unitary frameworks, by virtue of the essential normality
of the adjustment period that adolescence presents for the
individual and his social world. Thus, simple a priori
assumptions about particular problem aetiology, whether as
individual or social pathology, are inappropriate. How-

ever, the abiding social work principle of concern for the
client-in-his-situation does not, of itself, offer any help in
distinguishing causation for the purpose of deciding on
effective helping action. Meyer's (1976) conception of the
field of social work is useful in this respect. Her context, contours and content remind us of the dynamic and
relative nature of need, along a continuum from individual
need to social problem, becoming translated into social
policy. Thus the social worker should have an important
feedback function in shaping social policy and, in order to
carry it out as effectively as the function of helping with
particular needs, he must have a wider knowledge base than
has been considered necessary hitherto. In social work
with adolescents that feedback function, in order to be most
effective, would also need to be linked to those of other
relevant professionals, such as educationalists and youth
workers who operate more exclusively at the general needs
end of Meyer's continuum. It is in the middle area of that
continuum where the pooling of resources, both human and
material, is likely to be of the greatest significance for
social work organization, implying a flexibility across professional and departmental boundaries which is as yet uncommon.

Middleman and Goldberg's (1973) conception of the scope
of social work activity reflects this same principle of concern for the individual and the social situation. Their
model specifically proposes a division, by social work
specialization, between work at the different ends of the
continuum, i.e. between that primarily concerned with particular problems and that concerned with general needs.
Applied to the needs of adolescents, Middleman and Goldberg's model immediately suggests the usefulness of having
specialist social workers with adolescents in social services departments, capable of making the external links
mentioned above, as well as operating independently of, but
in close association with, their own referrals-based workers. To do so effectively, however, would imply specialization at area team level rather than higher in the organization as is sometimes the case.

The difficulties inherent in social work practice in dealing with both ends of Meyer's continuum become increasingly clear in using the unitary frameworks. The challenge
is how to organize a social work service that is at once
capable of responding to the particular and individual need,
of monitoring the pattern of individual needs to judge where

they move along the continuum towards social needs, and of
detecting and responding to those general needs which may
not be apparent from the referrals pattern. That challenge
is inherent also in the systems frameworks offered by Goldstein (1973) and by Pincus and Minahan (1973 and 1977), for,
although their illustrations start from single hypothetical
cases (i.e. from referrals-based work), the range of involvement in, and intervention with systems other than, the
single client raises questions about the feasibility of the
traditional organization of referrals-based work, and of
the relatively haphazard allocation of cases to caseloads of
wholly 'generic' social workers (see DHSS, 1978). The
implication of their models is that a wide range of methods
and levels of intervention can and should be available to be
used with appropriate other systems. Recent evidence and
discussion suggests that the answer may lie in the better
use of the social work team, mentioned earlier in the context of social learning, moving as Evans (1978) puts it, from
'individualized' team work to 'joint' team work, or from the
tennis to the football team concept. There has recently
been a growing and encouraging number of accounts appearing in the social work press of various attempts by social
work teams to move in this direction. Techniques such as
the Operational Priority System have been found valuable
in this respect and, importantly too, as a means of monitoring referrals patterns to detect trends in social needs
(Hall, 1975). But trends in social needs may not always be
reflected in referrals. For example, it is frequently the
case in rural areas that referrals tend to be clustered
around the urban centres where the social work agencies
are found, but it would be dangerous to assume that no
social welfare needs or problems exist in the more outlying
areas. Community workers normally work from outside
the agency rather than from within, and can thus provide an
essential element to the monitoring of social needs, as can
other non referrals-based professionals such as youth
workers. This would indicate the further development of
the generic social work team to include a variety of specialists from a broader social welfare field (as is beginning
to happen with the introduction of community workers), including both professional and para-professional elements.
   The unitary frameworks essentially link the different
approaches implicit in truly generic social work. Social
work of all kinds can then be seen as a craft, with the self
as a tool, the relationship as the medium and social learn-

ing as the product, elements which are as valid for youth work, adult education work and community work, for example, as they are for the more traditional forms of social work. Finally, the client or adolescent and his situation, that dynamic configuration, can be brought together into a manageable but still dynamic conceptualization by the very simple notion of a system.

Chapter four

Conflict and competence in inter-professional communication in the services for adolescents

Jack Dunham

/The previous papers have begun to emphasise the need to see adolescents in their social context, and to explore all the resources that may be available to them. Many of these resources, however, are not controlled by social workers, but are the responsibility of other professionals, such as school teachers and doctors. One of the tasks for social workers, therefore, may be to communicate and work with these other professionals on behalf of adolescents. This chapter explores and explains some of the problems in inter-professional communication and co-operation, and suggests ways of reducing these difficulties. It also stresses the need to see social work in the context of a range of resources available to young people, and therefore builds upon the interactional theme already developed in the previous two chapters. The ability to effectively collaborate with other professions, and with those within one's discipline who have a different ideology or practice preference, is crucial to good social work. Hence this chapter provides an essential background for the intervention chapters which follow./

Major problems of communication and co-operation between the professional workers who are involved in the education, social and medical services for adolescents are frequently reported. The reports mainly consist of anecdotal observations, but they have recently been supported by research studies whose methodology can be accepted with some degree of confidence. These problems appear to be caused to some extent by considerable isolation in professional training which may lead to an ignorance of the aims, procedures and role boundaries of other professional workers.

Difficulties in inter-professional understanding are frequently strongly reinforced by a continuing process of professionalisation after qualification when professional group
loyalties are emphasised.

The reports demand our attention because there are two
important consequences of these problems. The first is the
ineffective and often wasteful use of scarce resources for
adolescents. The second important consideration is concerned with the effects of the difficulties in communications
and co-operation on the professional workers who are responsible for providing the services for adolescents. These
are good grounds for analysing the possible causes and consequences of poor inter-professional communications and
for discussing the attempts which have been made to promote
more effective co-operation. As a framework for this
chapter I would like to consider three question:

1 What are the causes of the communications problems between the 'helping professions' concerned with adolescents' problems?
2 What are the consequences of these difficulties in
   inter-professional co-operation for the adolescents and
   their helpers?
3 What recommendations might be made to promote a more
   effective co-ordination of the available resources by
   reducing these difficulties?

THE CAUSES OF DIFFICULTIES IN INTER-PROFESSIONAL COMMUNICATIONS

Five major causes of these problems have been identified.
They are closely related to important differences between
the helping professions in education, training and experience. These influences are responsible for conflicts in
priorities, differences in language, restricted professional
perspectives, role conflict, and problems in sharing confidential information.

Conflicts in priorities

I have observed these differences during in-service training courses of social workers, educational welfare officers
and teachers. The EWOs reported difficult relationships
with social workers which were the result of differences in

priorities between the two agencies when they were dealing
with the same family. The main concern of the EWO, which
was returning a pupil to school, was often in conflict with
the work of the social worker who was working with the
family as a whole. The EWOs also reported important differences in status between themselves and other agencies
which results from the EWOs' lack of training.

The differences in the significance which social workers
and the members of other services attribute to their various
tasks can also be seen in the statement of the deputy headmaster of a comprehensive school made during one of my
Staff Development Conferences:

I am most concerned about girls who become pregnant
whilst still of compulsory school age. The lack of information on abortions often makes our job more difficult.
The attitude of Social Services towards girls who have
and keep their babies is to say that the baby comes first
and the girl must look after it - never mind school. By
law they are obliged to see that the girl continues her
education full time.

Differences in language

Professional training imparts a conceptual framework and a
language which are shared by people training in the same
disciplines but not by 'outsiders'. The concepts and the
language used to express them are often used as indications
of group membership and as a 'passport' to acceptance.
Entrance to the group is restricted to those who know the
language. Terms such as 'defence mechanisms', 'ration-
alisation', 'interpretation' and 'introjection' may be used as
an indication of special training and knowledge. The 'restricted' language is often dismissed as 'jargon' by the members of other groups. An attempt to communicate by using a
'general' code has been reported by a psychiatrist:

In practice, I find that a great deal of psycho-jargon can
be dispensed with to the benefit of patient and practitioner
alike. The majority of psychiatric work involves emi-
nently understandable misery and there is no need to use
terms like 'depression', 'neurotic' and 'psychopathy'
when homelier words like 'unhappiness', 'anxiety' and
'undesirable personality traits' will often - though not
always - do as well (Brewer, 1975, p. 15).
Goldberg and Neill (1972) have indicated another linguis-

tic difficulty which is the result of the same word having
different meanings when it is used by different professions.
They argue that 'urgent' and 'chronic' have very different
meanings in medicine and social work because doctors when
treating 'urgent cases' expect action to be taken within
hours, while social workers often think that more time is
needed to assess the factors involved:

> In such cases as compulsory admission to a mental hospi-
> tal, when doctors may expect rapid action, they may find
> that social workers wish to proceed more cautiously, and
> to spend time assessing the total situation. Doctors may
> then accuse social workers of confusing action on medical
> grounds with psychological or social factors which they
> regard as irrelevant. Equally, many social workers are
> more aware than doctors of the social and emotional han-
> dicaps which can occur when individuals become institu-
> tionalised. They will try as far as possible to avoid re-
> moving them from their families and the community (Gold-
> berg and Neill, 1972, p. 150).

Restricted professional perspectives

These conceptual and linguistic differences which begin in
the initial training courses are reinforced by the development of professional group loyalties. This process begins
when a newly qualified professional worker joins his professional group. The effects of professionalisation are:

(a) Each professional group approaches a client's treat-
     ment from the point of view of its own professional per-
     spectives, which it believes to be the best available.
(b) Differences exist between the groups in their explana-
     tions of how clients' difficulties come about. Whether
     such difficulties stem mainly from constitutional factors
     or from environmental influences is often an area of
     deep disagreement.
(c) The ignorance of another profession's purposes and
     procedures are major stumbling-blocks to co-operation.
(d) An unawareness of the effects of professionalisation
     can lead to an inability to understand its restrictive
     consequences; for example, psychologists, social
     workers and psychiatrists use such terms as 'mature'
     or 'emotionally stable' as if there was general agree-
     ment about their meaning. They often seem unable to
     understand why they appear to be so narrow and rigid
     in the eyes of their colleagues.

Role-conflict

These criticisms of restricted professional perspectives
are supported by some recent entrants to the 'helping' professions, as for instance in social work where the newly
trained may be very critical of the traditional diagnostic
categories of mental illness used by their older colleagues,
or their attitudes towards medication and mental hospitals.
In the Probation and After-Care Service the differences
between experienced officers and the recently qualified are
similarly wide and significant. A report by a probation
officer on one of my in-service training courses gives further details of the effects of these differences:

> It may be helpful to look at the growing pains of an ex-
> panding Probation and After-Care Service, and in the
> expectations of its new and older members. The dif-
> fering attitudes of officers from a variety of back-
> grounds and training courses, some more generic,
> probably means a less uniform approach to the work,
> which is likely to be the cause of conflict within a group
> or office. Relationships with other social services,
> particularly the Social Services Department, and with
> local government and the lack of understanding between
> ourselves and with them are also sources of stress

Problems in sharing confidential information

The question of confidentiality presents considerable problems for close professional co-operation. Doctors and
social workers are often reluctant to share their information with other professional workers, and co-operation with
them is hindered. But the claims of confidentiality can be
used as an effective weapon in inter-group conflict by the
withholding of information. The criterion of other agencies' 'need-to-know' is replaced by the self-protective
barrier of restricted information sharing.
    These problems of sharing confidential information,
role conflict, restricted professional perspectives, differences in language, and conflicts in priorities have significant implications for adolescents and the professional
workers who are attempting to provide effective services
for them.

THE EFFECTS OF INTER-PROFESSIONAL COMMUNICA-
TION PROBLEMS ON SERVICES FOR ADOLESCENTS

Poor inter-professional communications have unfavourable
consequences for the effectiveness of the services which
should benefit adolescents.   Some of these effects may be
seen in the reports of inadequate co-operation between
Education, Welfare and Social Services Departments.   One
report which provides a good example of the unhelpful
effects of an isolationalist approach to young people's problems was prepared for a Staff Development Conference
which I organised in a comprehensive school:

> Shirley is 14.   Her school records show intermittent
> incidents of difficult behaviour from the beginning of
> junior school onwards.   Towards the end of the second
> year in secondary school her disturbed spells became
> more frequent and were often marked by a tendency to be
> insolent to teachers, in particular to men.   At the begin-
> ning of the third year the situation deteriorated and she
> had substantial periods of truancy.   When in school,
> Shirley was frequently abusive to teachers.   Her mother
> was invited to school and she informed the year head that
> she had recently left her husband, taking Shirley as well
> as an older son by her previous marriage.   Her atten-
> dance improved but she was increasingly disturbed in
> school.   About six weeks after the interview with her
> mother, Shirley ran away from home.   Her half-brother
> found her the next day and brought her home without any
> difficulty.   Mother spoke to the year head on the phone,
> but the school received very little information about the
> incident.
>
> A week later Shirley found her mother dead at the
> bottom of the stairs in her house.   It was reported at the
> inquest that she had been an alcoholic for some years.
> Shirley went to live with her father, and in school her
> behaviour deteriorated sharply.
>
> At that point the form teacher and year head met with
> the headmaster to discuss the situation.   They felt that
> although they had considerable sympathy for the girl in
> these circumstances, they had a responsibility to the
> other children.   The policy from then on was to be firm
> with Shirley.   This decision was discussed with the
> father.   He said that he had also started by making
> allowances but had come to the conclusion that he must be
> more strict.

> There was some improvement in Shirley's behaviour,
> but she still had violent outbursts in which she was ex-
> tremely abusive to members of staff. They began to
> complain about the disruption caused to their lessons and
> the hurt caused them by Shirley's abusive tongue. She
> was sent out of a lesson for disruption and the head sus-
> pended her.

It seems probable that Shirley will not be helped to solve
her problem until a wider view is taken of the nature of her
difficulties. This change in perspective is unlikely to
develop until a more comprehensive inter-professional
approach is used, and thus more helpful understanding is
being blocked by strong barriers to co-operation and communication between the 'caring' professions.

The effects of poor communications on the identification
of adolescents' difficulties can also be seen in a study by
Gay, Copus and Holder (1973) of maladjusted children in
Bristol. This research was concerned with the work of a
community mental health team which included psychologists,
psychiatrists, school medical officers, a social worker and
teachers. The differences between psychiatrists and
teachers in the diagnosis of maladjustment in a comprehensive school was one of the main themes of the investigation.
A sample of the pupils was assessed by their teachers on
the Bristol Social Adjustment Guide (Stott, 1966) and by the
psychiatrists who used Rutter's psychiatric interviews
technique (Rutter and Graham, 1968). Gay, Copus and
Holder concluded in their report:

> There was psychiatric confirmation of 'psychiatric abnor-
> mality' in 64.2% of the children who were assessed by
> their teachers as 'maladjusted'. A further group of
> children (26.9%) who were seen by their teachers as
> 'stable' were identified by the psychiatrists as suffering
> from psychiatric abnormality. The teaching staff tended
> to identify the acting-out-boys - who were not identified
> as maladjusted by the psychiatrists - the psychiatrists
> were much more concerned with the withdrawn, depres-
> sed girls who were seen by their teachers as 'stable' -
> since they were not presenting any problems in class
> (Gay, Copus and Holder, 1973).

If these differences in diagnostic criteria of the psychiatrists and teachers are not reduced by good inter-professional communications and co-operation, both the disruptive boys and the depressed girls may not receive adequate
support as they attempt to identify and cope with their
problems.

These adverse consequences of communication difficulties
between the different services concerned with mental health
have also been reported by Kenny and Whitehead:

Any rapid and effective communication between separate
but interdependent branches can expect occasional problems, but the health services in general and the psychiatric services in particular seem to develop more than
their fair share of them. These problems affecting the
progress and outcome of a mental disorder arise directly
from failures of communications between the branches.
Some of the more common difficulties for patients and
relatives are listed below. In a different field of work
they might be called demarcation disputes. Two examples
are:

(i) The family doctor and some social workers disagree
about the nature of the patient's problem. Each of
them pursues his own line of intervention to the be-
wilderment of the patient. (This situation can apply
with any combination of the three professionals involved – family doctor, psychiatrist and social
worker.)

(ii) The psychiatrist does not refer any patient to local
authority social workers because he cannot control
their activities and uses nurses instead for all
follow-up work, whether or not they are appropriate
people for the job. The overall effect of these situations is to make the patient and his family feel that
they are being treated like parcels rather than
people

(Kenny and Whitehead, 1974, p. 97).

The significance of inter-professional communications
barriers between hospital and community services can also
be seen in the report of a psychiatrist who is the Director
of the Brent Consultation Centre. A boy aged 17 who had
attempted to commit suicide had been referred to him:

Bill sought help at the suggestion of his family doctor.
He had recently been discharged from hospital after
having made a serious suicide attempt. The doctor had
hoped that Bill would be kept in hospital for a period when
he might be offered psychiatric treatment but instead he
was discharged three days after having been admitted.
He had taken seventy aspirins and was found in bed semi-
conscious by his father. Bill's parents were quite ready
to take the advice of friends to 'forget about it' – but the
family doctor insisted that something must be done to help

him, feeling that without treatment Bill was at risk of killing himself. I agree with the doctor (Laufer, 1975, p. 88).

These reports provide support for the claims which have been made recently by Fitzherbert (1977) and Jones (1977) that there are serious consequences for children and adolescents when the helping professions cannot communicate effectively with each other and are unsuccessful in inter-professional co-operation. These reports also indicate that there are significant effects on the professional workers themselves.

The effects of communications problems on professional workers

Communications difficulties are reported as major causes of stress by workers in the 'caring' professions. In my exploratory studies with residential social workers (Dunham, 1978) I asked them to report on their stress situations and stress responses (see also Chapter eight). Their written reports indicated that communication difficulties were common causes of stress for them. They complained to me of a lack of liaison with the management hierarchy in Social Services and of management's poor understanding of the role of residential social workers.

The responses of staff to these stress situations can be grouped into three main categories: behavioural, emotional and psychosomatic. Appley and Trumbull (1967) have proposed a framework of 'thresholds' which individuals pass through as they react to stress situations of increasing severity. These stages are (i) new behaviour, (ii) frustration, (iii) anxiety, (iv) psychosomatic symptoms, and (v) exhaustion.

New behaviour is developed in response to the recognition of demands which may lead to the development of additional professional skills. This is the new coping behaviour threshold. If these skills are unsuccessful the frustrations threshold is reached. If there is a continuing failure to cope the worker may begin to doubt his competence to meet these demands and he will experience strong feelings of anxiety. More severe disturbances may follow which may be accompanied by psychosomatic symptoms. As the individual uses up his coping resources he will reach the stage of exhaustion.

All these stages and thresholds are experienced by residential workers. Their reports also indicate some responses which are outside Appley and Trumbull's framework.
These are withdrawal, displaced aggression, defensive
reactions and depression.

Some of these responses can be noted in the reports of
three heads of Children's Homes on their relationships with
field social workers. One of them reported:

My main stress situation is the peculiar people I work
with i.e. field social workers. I had to go to Lancashire
with two social workers to discuss whether two boys in
my care were to be allowed to return to their father when
he was released from prison. The care committee decided against it. All the way back I was wondering how to
tell the boys. The social workers were doing a cross-
word. I was nearly sick with anger at their behaviour.

The second report was concerned with the effects of poor
communications in relation to policy changes:

Social Services are trying to push kids onto me who I
think should not be here, e.g. last week it was a maladjusted fifteen year old girl who was having a sexual relationship with a fairground worker. My criterion is that
this is a long-stay Children's Home and I must think
whether this girl will fit into the Home, i.e. with care
staff and domestic staff and the other boys and girls.
There always seems to be a crisis in placing a child. I
want a change in the designation of the Home to signify
our changed roles which require changes in the residential workers' skills. There are considerable differences between long-stay care needs and crisis care needs.

The third warden's report referred to problems in decision-
making:

When their father died the children were taken into care
and placed in our Home. The mother who had left the
family four years earlier now contacted Social Services
and said that she wanted to remove the children from the
Home immediately so that they would live with her. She
was living with a man and his three children. In my
opinion it was necessary to assess the mother's ability
and willingness to care for nine children before we
agreed to her demands. The social worker, who was
supported by her superiors, appeared to be unaware of
the apparent dangers in this situation. Conflict arose
between the field worker and myself about the decisions
which were required.

These reports are blatantly one sided and make no attempt to understand the field social workers' reactions. Residential social workers are sometimes responsible for difficulties in communications with social services because of the barriers which they develop around their Homes. They may do this by belittling the importance of field social workers to their residents and by restricting the opportunities which field social workers need to interview young people in the Homes.

Some of the frustrations of field social workers are discussed in an account of the effects of poor communications between social workers and doctors in a report to the Standing Joint Liaison Committee between the British Association of Social Workers and the Royal College of General Practitioners:

Inter-professional hostility, which may be based on misunderstanding and feelings of mutual frustration and impatience, interferes with constructive collaboration. Inadequate or distorted communication often means that general practitioners and social workers are either both working separately with the same individual or that neither is working with the person in need, because each is waiting for the other to take the first step. Failure to know of the other's involvement (or lack of it), or failure to report progress or change in the situation, can be a source of endless irritation to both professions. Failure to see the relevance of the other's role or the need for his expertise in certain situations can lead to hostility and conflict (Ratoff, Rose and Smith, 1974, p. 86).

The effects of conflict in inter-professional relationships between teachers and the staff of a Child Guidance Clinic have been examined by Skynner (1974). His clinic team – psychiatrist, psychologist, psychiatric social workers and child psycho-therapist – visited a comprehensive school every month for two years to discuss with the staff the pupils who were problems in the school. Skynner discusses the contact and interaction between the teachers and the clinic team as the experiment progressed:

At our first meeting there was a large attendance, perhaps about 30 teachers in all. There may have been a feeling among the teachers that the large group situation was too chaotic because the senior staff altered the arrangements for our second visit without prior agreement or warning. Only four teachers were present and it was explained to us that they were the only ones con-

cerned in the case.   The third visit brought a crisis.
We arrived on time to find the library, where we held our
meetings, locked, while the teachers were still eating
and paid little attention to our presence.   We were late
starting and exactly as the session was due to end, a
second case was raised which took us ten minutes over
our time (Skynner, 1974, p. 103).
Gradually the teachers' confidence in the team's contributions increased.   But this development was not continuous:
A marked advance would often be followed by a partial
regression, a well attended and lively session by late-
ness, absence and seemingly unrewarding interchange.
In one session we found ourselves once again locked out,
the teachers eating; almost everyone was late, with no
excuses made; and the discussion of cases seemed incon-
clusive and marked by indifference and fragmentation with
people often talking together in two's or three's (Skynner,
1974, p. 110).
These reports of the stress which is caused by communication problems indicate the importance of trying to support
the professional workers as they attempt to care for adolescents.   This is a complex area because there are so many
possible problems.   But the fact that stress is an additional
barrier to inter-professional co-operation, as well as a
consequence of communications difficulties, is a strong incentive to explore different models of inter-professional
co-operation.

THE IMPROVEMENT OF COMMUNICATIONS AND CO-OPERATION

Some major tasks in the improvement of inter-professional
communication have been set out in the working paper produced by the Institute of Organisation and Social Studies at
Brunel University (1976) in which a number of crucial questions are asked:
How can better working links be established between
various practitioners, for example, doctors, nurses and
social workers who are concerned in the same cases?
How can better communication patterns be established
and better co-ordination and continuity be achieved?
Brunel University, 1976, p. 7).
There is a strong belief amongst professional workers
that communications will be improved by means of contact

between the members of different professional groups. Unfortunately some forms of interaction may not be very helpful and it is important to examine, rather than to accept, the assumption that more contacts will improve communications.

Contact in case-conferences

The experiences which members have in case-conferences may reinforce their perception of intransigent fellow-professionals who are jealous of their professional boundaries. When I worked in a Child Guidance Clinic I was very aware in the weekly case-conferences of the expectations from my colleagues to keep within my psychologist's role and only to present information about intelligence, attainments, attitudes and personality.

Bland has also perceived these sensitive boundaries in case-conferences:

> On some occasions when case conferences have taken place with nursing staff, it has been obvious that the charge nurse has felt himself to be under assessment, and has ignored the value other professionals placed on his contribution. I have found that however good the relationship being built up, the merest breath of criticism is sufficient to reveal concealed or repressed antagonisms (Bland, 1976).

Contact in joint in-service training

The contact which is experienced in joint in-service training courses may not be any more helpful in modifying unfavourable stereotypes. In the last three years I have organised two joint courses for teachers and social workers concerned with socially disadvantaged children and adolescents. These conferences revealed considerable differences, not only in the perspectives of these groups of professional workers towards disadvantaged children and adolescents, but also toward each other. The teachers thought that the social workers paid too much attention to home and community factors and not enough to what could be done in school. The social workers thought that the teachers largely ignored the significance of factors outside the school. Inter-disciplinary co-operation may not have been fostered by this experience which may have instead confirmed the stereotypes each group had of the other one.

However during a joint training exercise between postgraduate medical and social work students there was evidence of changing, and more positive, inter-professional perceptions, but this was only after open and frank discussions between the professionals involved (Pritchard, Taylor and King, 1978).

Working parties

The favourable effects of a more intensive form of contact have been reported by Payne (1976).   This is an account of the setting-up of a working party composed of twelve GPs, social workers and health visitors in Southampton.   Payne reported that this group sparked off an awareness of the need for better co-operation and understanding between the professions so that gradually there evolved a 'flourishing network of sub-groups and liaison schemes which now provide regular opportunities for shared learning and decision making'.

The effect of working parties on the interactions between teachers and social workers was the main focus of a large-scale project, which was carried out between 1975 and 1977 in South Wales.   It consisted of almost 200 people representing all the services concerned with children which were provided through central and local government and by voluntary organisations in South Glamorgan.   The project was set up because of the concern that had been expressed by the caring professions in this area about the problems of children and their families, particularly in the context of education, juvenile offending, truancy and social disadvantage.   This project consisted of multi-disciplinary working groups which met regularly in residential and day 'meetings' to consider communication difficulties between teachers and social workers and to make recommendations to reduce these difficulties.   Their reports have been edited by Kahan (1977) and they show that some of these recommendations are already in operation:

> Monthly meetings between heads of schools and social
> work teams have been established in some areas and
> monthly meetings between social workers, heads of
> junior schools, education welfare officers and health
> visitors are being held at the local health centre
> (Kahan, 1977, p. 120).

The reports also claimed that some clarification of their
respective roles had been achieved by the different professional workers in the project, though it was not stated by
the writers how these changes in perception had been
assessed.

Some of the results of the project indicated that role
clarification does not necessarily mean better co-operation:

There was a great deal of conflict during the early meetings and members withdrew into their respective 'corners'. The working group then divided into sub-groups
although this had initially been rejected by the total group
(ibid., p. 121).

There was, however, general agreement amongst the reports of the working groups of the role of the EWO:

The education welfare officer is seen as crucial, a key
person, though at present undervalued. He liaises with
other agencies including housing and social services and
he could be designated the liaison officer in schools
(ibid., p. 122).

The role of the liaison officer/negotiator

Liaison and negotiation roles are crucial in improving contact between different professions. For instance, Skynner's attempts to improve inter-professional communications
between comprehensive school teachers and the staff of a
Child Guidance Clinic by regular discussions of disruptive
pupil behaviour over a two-year period have been referred
to earlier in the chapter. He reported that at the end of
the experiment there appeared to have been a reduction in
inter-group conflict and stereotyping and the development of
good professional relationships:

Staff spoke of the ability they now had to share problems
and communicate about them as well as the confidence they
now possessed that they would cope. It was, however,
impossible to decide how much our meetings had contributed to this improvement (Skynner, 1974, p. 114).

The contributions of the educational psychologist to the
maintenance of good communications appear to have been
very important. Skynner reports that 'He frequently
played a vital role in linking us, perceiving what difficulties of communication there might be and clarifying the difficulties of each side to the other' (ibid., p. 113). This
is an excellent definition not only of the role of a psycholo-

gist in a school staff – clinic team experiment but of the role
of a negotiator in a whole range of inter-group situations.
The analysis of the significant differences in perception
which doctors, nurses, teachers, social workers have of
each others' roles, and which often lead to frustration and
anger, is an important contribution by a negotiator in the
reduction of communication barriers, and even within a professional group there can be confusion and disagreement
over role definition (Pritchard and Taylor, 1979).

The importance of the negotiator role can be noted also
in the account which the Head of a South London comprehensive school wrote of the development of a sound preventive
service for the adolescents in her school. Here the role
was played by the school-based social worker:

> We recognise that though teachers can do a great deal to
> help pupils 'at risk' by the way they teach, by providing
> a 'model' of adult behaviour, by listening to and support-
> ing the pupil, there is a need for specialist help to be
> brought in at the earliest opportunity if an effective pre-
> ventative (rather than remedial) service is to be provided.
> Attached to the first year (age 11-12) we have a school-
> based social worker seconded full-time from social ser-
> vices, working closely with the head of year, form tutor
> and education welfare officer. For the rest of the school
> we have appointed our own part-time counsellor and
> social worker. Not only are the pupils helped directly
> through these services, but the teachers too can get
> 'instant' advice and support.
>
> Teachers are less tempted to get out of role, yet their
> skills are not lost, rather enhanced. The boundaries be-
> tween the professions are not blurred, yet the amount of
> direct help to the pupils is increased, and referrals to
> specialists can be made early enough to be effective
> (Jones, 1976, p. 22).

Pritchard and Butler (1978) have contributed further evidence of the usefulness of the role of negotiator in a study
of the response to school phobia and truancy of a sample of
teachers in secondary schools. The authors found significant differences in the teachers' responses between the
schools with a Youth Tutor and those who did not have one.
The teachers in the Youth Tutor schools were more 'therapeutically orientated' towards the school phobia and truancy
and it was claimed that these developments had occurred because, 'The work of the Youth Tutor clearly makes an impression upon his colleagues in that they conceptualise prob-

lems in a much more comprehensive fashion which in turn
appears to positively influence the ethos of the school'
(Pritchard and Butler, 1978, p. 280).

It might be thought that these differences were due to the
variation of head teachers, with the 'sympathetic' head-
teachers appointing Youth Tutors. In fact this was not the
case – a feature which was noted by the senior administra-
tors of the LEA involved. Perhaps the most encouraging
aspect of the 'negotiator' role was found by Rose and Marshall (1974). Their controlled and matched study of secondary schools found that those schools with social workers
or counsellors attached had statistically significantly
lower delinquency and higher attendance rates than schools
without such staff. An important secondary outcome was
the noticeably 'better communications' within the schools.

The contribution of teamwork

There is also some evidence that attitudes are changed and
conflict is reduced by inter-professional teamwork. The
essential condition is that the members must accept the
necessity of working together because their tasks cannot be
accomplished by individuals or groups working separately.
These common tasks have been called 'superordinate goals'
by Sherif (1967) because 'they have a compelling appeal for
members of each group, but which neither group can
achieve without the participation of the other.' Sherif
arranged a series of experiments to test his hypothesis that
these goals would reduce inter-group conflict. For instance:

> One day the two groups of boys in the camp went on an
> outing at a lake some distance away. A large truck was
> to go for food. But when everyone was hungry and ready
> to eat, it developed that the truck would not start (the
> staff of the camp had taken care of that). The boys got
> a rope – which they had previously used in their acrimon-
> ious tug-of-war – and all pulled together to start the
> truck (Sherif, 1967).

Sherif reported that single situations did not dispel the
inter-group hostility. A series of activities requiring interdependent action was required before co-operation
started to replace competition. He was also aware of the
need to verify these small-scale experiments in different
settings to test their relevance for a wider range of inter-

group conflict situations. These attempts are discussed in
detail in his book, and provide support for his claims that
the acceptance of superordinate goals can lead to the reduction of inter-group conflict in industrial organisations.

The relevance of Sherif's concept for the improvement of
inter-professional teamwork in the services for adolescents
should also be considered. Some reports which I have received are encouraging. One was made to me by the
teacher in a special unit in a comprehensive school when I
asked him to identify the sources of support in his work:

> In our situation we are very lucky in having a very good
> support team. This I feel to be essential. (Our team
> consists of a psychiatrist, psychologist and social
> worker.) We also have opportunities to meet staff who
> work in similar situations and face similar problems to
> our own at meetings held two or three times each term.

The second report, which was made by the Head of a
Community Home in which one of my students was working,
emphasised the importance of different professional groups
supporting each other instead of remaining in positions of
unproductive conflict. He argued that inter-professional
communication and co-operation can be improved if common
concerns can be found in which different professionals can
share.

These brief reports indicate the importance of competence in multi-disciplinary teamwork skills in the organisation of an integrated service for adolescents (see also
Chapter eight). They suggest that the identification and
development of these skills should have an important place
in research projects and initial and in-service training.

SUMMARY

There are major problems of communications and co-operation between the workers who are professionally concerned
with adolescents. These problems are caused by differences in priorities and language, and by ignorance of the aims
and procedures amongst the people who should be working
together to provide an integrated service. There are barriers to the necessary flow of information between the
workers because of caution over confidentiality, and on
account of strong professional group loyalties.

Better links between doctors, nurses, teachers, social
workers, policemen, psychologists and probation officers

can be developed but not necessarily in case-conferences or
joint training courses at the in-service level. There is
evidence that communication barriers can be reduced if the
workers acknowledge the necessity of working together to
identify and achieve common tasks. The skills of working
in an integrated manner include the development of a shared
language, and understanding how to conduct the process of
negotiating. These skills can be learned by all professional workers who want to achieve the 'superordinate goal' of
improving the services for adolescents.

Part II

Social work
with adolescents

Chapter five

Counselling the adolescent
and his family

Audrey Taylor and Colin Pritchard

/Having explored in Part I of the book some general themes
about adolescence and social work, the text now focuses in
more detail upon social work intervention with and for adolescents. Taylor and Pritchard begin by discussing some of
the issues which arise in the family, and examine some of
the tasks and techniques relevant for the social worker in
counselling the adolescent and his parents. The counselling skills and approaches discussed and illustrated in this
chapter may well be required of any practitioner who has
direct contact with young people and their parents. This
approach is relevant to both residential and fieldwork settings, and irrespective of whether the primary or initial
mode of intervention is seen as casework, groupwork or
community work._/

Social work with adolescents implies for us direct face-to-
face contact with young people. This often involves the
adolescent and his family in a process of counselling. To
explore adequately a counselling approach we first need to
re-examine, albeit briefly, some of the key areas of adolescent and family development already discussed by Dunham
and Jones in Chapter two. This will allow us to relate
more directly the discussion of assessment to the description of some counselling responses. The detailing of
issues which may occur for many adolescents and their
parents helps us to consider more readily typical family and
individual responses to stress, and to decide when these
reactions are unhelpful or pathological.

The classic model of adolescence has been one of 'storm
and stress', through which most adolescents had to pass.
Recently, however, there has been a major reconsideration

of such ideas, so that Rutter (1976) poses the question: 'Is adolescent turmoil fact or fiction?' He examines evidence drawn from a wide range of studies and suggests that, although parents and adolescents may quite commonly disagree about such matters as dress, hair length and staying out late, parent-child 'alienation' is relatively rare unless the adolescent is already showing some psychiatric problems; however, perhaps as many as 50 per cent of adolescents experience feelings of self-doubt and misery. He concludes that adolescent turmoil is a fact, but that its psychiatric importance has been exaggerated in the past.

Numerous recent studies, based upon large samples drawn from 'non-pathological' groups, support Rutter's conclusions (Masterson, 1967; Offer and Offer, 1969; King, 1972). On the other hand Nuttall et al. (1977) from the USA, and Cerny (1977) from Europe, found that many adolescents welcome advice and counselling on a range of transient problems of a psycho-social nature, and benefit from a counselling service that is objective and informed. Both these studies discovered that approximately 25 per cent of youngsters have difficulties of moderate complexity requiring medium-term help. Estimates of moderate 'maladjustment' amongst 12- to 16-year-olds in the UK tend to be around 15-18 per cent, with the prevalence of severe problems ranging between 3 and 7 per cent (Pringle, 1967; Gath et al., 1977). As there are approximately 4,000,000 school children within the adolescent age range, a conservative estimate of problems, i.e. 3 per cent, yields a figure of about 120,000. Not surprisingly, the professional tends to concentrate upon the most problematic group; but should more attention be given to the much larger group with moderately severe problems, as suggested by Nuttall et al.?

In our consideration of the adolescent and his family we take for granted the influence of the socio-political context in which families live; but, as space precludes examination of these macro social factors, we will concentrate upon the systems which immediately impinge upon the family. Equally it is recognised that some adolescents do not live with their families, and that they will, therefore, be faced with additional pressures in the resolution of the normal 'crisis' of adolescent development.

One very significant factor we would wish to stress is that adolescence often coincides with the parents' 'mid-life crisis'. Just as adolescents are having to adjust to their new role, so parents are having to adjust to their middle years. For both parents and children these developmental tasks are undertaken in a socio-cultural setting which is subject to constant change. Parents' own experience of adolescence offers little guide with regard to values or norms. They can be genuinely confused as to what they should or should not do in their role as parents, or about what is 'normal' behaviour for adolescents. The present for adolescents is by definition normal and they may find their parents' attitudes quite inexplicable (Davies, 1974).

There is an innate competitiveness between parents and adolescents. In their eagerness to assert their own identity, adolescents often challenge their parents' attainments, standards and behaviour, pouring scorn on them as being 'old', 'past it' and 'out-of-date'. Parents may feel compelled to assert themselves in return and some, indeed, seem to experience almost a second adolescence in their wish to prove their youth and sexual attractiveness.

The competitiveness may be further accentuated by the greater emphasis now being placed upon the self-realisation of the individual (Maslow, 1968; Rogers, 1962), so that parents feel justified in seeking self-fulfilment, rather than putting aside their own needs in favour of those of their child. This is a complex topic which we will be looking at in more detail later.

THE TASK OF THE ADOLESCENT

Anna Freud (1965) defined the primary task of the human child as being to develop into the mature and autonomous adult, thus linking biological and psycho-social approaches to human growth and development. Within this primary task we can locate two interlocking sub-tasks, namely, the development of an adult identity, and the achievement of independence in economic, social and emotional spheres. Growth implies change, and change is often painful and stressful to those concerned. One particular problem for both parents and adolescent is the adolescent's changeability, as he oscillates between the attractions of an independent identity and the security of remaining as he is within the protection of, and dependent upon, his family. Hindrances to growth and maturation may be located outside the family (Wilson, 1974), or may be found within earlier unresolved conflicts, which are reactivated as the

family experience the push and pull of the shared adolescent process (Josselyn, 1952). This process has been described as a time bomb, which is ticking away with a potential for an explosion which varies between an inconvenient 'pop' and a disruptive 'bang' (Pritchard and Taylor, 1978).
Support for this idea can be found in the work of Nuttall et al. (1977) and Cerny (1977) who list the problems and anxieties most frequently said by adolescents to concern them. These are in the spheres of identity creation and the establishment of independence, and they will be looked at more closely as we examine the adolescent task under the headings of emotional, social, economic and sexual aspects.

Emotional aspects

The adolescent seeks to resolve the issue of 'Who am I?' and of relationships with parents and other members of his family. This coincides with a spurt in cognitive ability (Mussen et al., 1974) which enables him for the first time to reflectively analyse his emotional experience.

Social aspects

Linked with family relationships are relationships with peers and his identification with his particular reference group. The norms of this group can on the one hand reassure by offering group acceptance, and on the other they can be disruptively competitive with parental and wider social standards. Later they can become a rigid parameter from which the adolescent must again make a move for independence (Erikson, 1977).

Economic aspects

The attractions of economic independence increase as the youngster meets the full flood of the market forces, which are exploitatively focused upon his age group. These attractions have to be balanced against those of future economic gain, and its present accompanying dependence upon parents, if the teenager is to continue in the role of pupil and student. Rutter (1976) suggests that there is evidence that such economic dependence brings with it increasing risk of estrangement between parent and child.

Sexual aspects

The major hormonal changes which result in the physical pressures of developing sexuality bring with them the additional pressure for the adolescent of having to present himself as a sexually attractive object to his peer group.
Many adults, including parents, fail to appreciate just how overwhelming sexual feelings can be at this period. It is coping with this very newness, and its accompanying ex-

citement and anxiety, that can present the adolescent with
such a formidable task.   Despite the lifting of traditional
taboos, sexual matters continue to arouse strong feelings
in all concerned, particularly parents, who may well find
it impossible to remain neutral in the face of the change in
the sexual status of their child.   This may prove a particular problem for the parents of handicapped children (see,
for instance, Craft and Craft, 1978).

THE TASK OF THE FAMILY

For some the family is the source of a questionable psychological orthodoxy (Cooper, 1971).   Yet copious literature
demonstrates the accepted centrality of the family as a
major determinant in shaping the individual's personality
and his perception of the world (Coser, 1974).   For these
writers the family is the basis for induction of concepts of
'normality' and the source of protection, affection and nur-
turing (Rutter, 1975).   This wide range of tasks may, in
part, account for the strengths and weaknesses that are to
be perceived in families.   The family group attempts to
meet the needs of all its members simultaneously, and thus
seeks to sustain a series of relationships that are at one
and the same time supportive and competitive.

   Society expects parents to put the child's interests first
(Goldstein et al., 1977).   When a young person becomes an
adolescent and begins to make 'adult-like' demands, such
altruism becomes more difficult.   We would suggest that
although altruism is an essential ingredient of 'good enough
parenting' (Winnicott, 1960; CCETSW, 1978) at every
stage of the parenting process, it needs to be balanced with
a degree of self interest.   Too great a degree of parental
self interest may mean a child lacking in care and support,
and too little may be productive of a child 'smothered' by
parents who value themselves only for their parenting role.
Such situations are particularly likely to lead to conflict
in adolescence as children struggle to escape the over-
tight constraints of their family whilst parents refuse to
accept that their role must change.

   We will now examine the task of the family along the same
lines as that of the adolescent, but considering the needs of
both parents and children.   In doing this we will begin to
highlight some of the normal flashpoints of family conflict.

Emotional aspects

For the adolescent, the family should be a source of emotional support because it can offer the experience of affection, approval and consistency (see Coser, 1974), and it can be an emotional refuge from which to explore and experience the wider adolescent world. For parents, the family needs to be a place of emotional comfort which may be seen as compensating them for frustrations in other areas of their lives and reaffirming their identity and worth in the face of diminution of physical prowess and sexual attractiveness, and of their increasing experience of personal loss, such as the death of their own parents.

A factor which contributes to feelings of self worth and competence in the early years of parenthood is the dependence of children, and their admiration of the superior knowledge and wisdom of their parents. It can be all the more difficult, therefore, for parents to cope with adolescent children who are now critical and attacking on many fronts. Equally it can be difficult for parents to cope with the change in the balance of power necessitated by their children's growth towards adulthood without totally abandoning any responsibility for establishing limits or boundaries.

The arrival of adolescence may represent a threat to women for whom motherhood is the most important role in life. Bart (1969 and 1971) suggests that some women at this time may develop a depressive illness. Certainly the 'empty nest syndrome' (Glick and Kessler, 1974) is well known to family therapists who remark upon the difficulties faced by parents at this stage in the family life-cycle. To many parents the prospect of 'paired singularity' is unwelcome, for it may involve a reassessment of the marital relationships, when conflicts which have been dormant for many years may re-emerge.

Differences in perspectives between parents and children are always a potential source of conflict. Parents, like Janus, look two ways – towards the past and towards the future; for them the adolescent symbolises continuity and perhaps a compensation for their own unsatisfactory childhood. For young people, often only the present is important, and they may bitterly resent the way in which parents appear to be planning their future for them.

Socio-economic aspects

The family, for parents, can be the apogee of social success or failure, a reflection of their achievements. To the

adolescent the family offers a place in which to establish a
social identity and develop appropriate social skills.   At
the same time the adolescent is supported by his parents,
and this is sometimes an unpalatable fact for him to accept.
The costs involved in caring for an adolescent are considerable.   In particular there are likely to be demands upon
parents for a wider range of clothes and entertainments
than previously.   These demands may lead to resentment
on the part of parents or to loss of status in the peer group
for an adolescent who cannot keep up with the accepted
norms of the group.

It should be remembered that for most women now over
the age of 35, educational, economic and social opportunities were severely limited.   For such mothers, the relatively greater opportunities open to their daughters may at
one level be a cause for satisfaction, while at another
level, serve only as a reminder of the opportunities which
have been denied them.

Sexual aspects

For the adolescent, the family has an important gender-
modelling role (Drake and McDougall, 1977).   For adults,
the marital relationship is expected to provide sexual satisfaction, comfort and constancy.   Parents' attitude to their
children's developing sexuality may be ambivalent.
Anxiety aroused by the instability of adolescent behaviour
may threaten parents' veneer of adjustment, and bring back
into consciousness aspects of themselves which they would
rather forget, e.g. previous sexual behaviour.   It is also
an area in which traditional values may be reasserted by
parents, especially in the case of daughters.

We have already referred to the emphasis currently being
placed upon the individual's right to self-realisation.   This
emphasis is clearly reflected in the changing attitudes to
marriage, so that, for example, the recent consultative
document issued by the Working Party on Marriage Guidance
(1979) comments that 'Personal development and satisfaction
are core values underlying contemporary expectations of
marriage.'   Where expectations are not realised, marital
partners may now be unwilling to continue in the relationship, with the consequence that many adolescents will be
affected by the separation, divorce and remarriage of their
parents, often in terms of stress and/or socio-economic
deprivation.   In 1976, for instance, 47,000 divorces took
place which also involved children aged 11-15 ('Social
Trends', 1979).

It would seem that stress in any of the four main areas
referred to above (i.e. emotional, social, economic or
sexual) is part of the normal process of the life-cycle
(Erikson, 1977; Rutter, 1976; see also Chapter two).
One other stress which impinges upon the family is the
problem of ill health, where acute illness, or chronic and
handicapping conditions, may affect the balance of family
functioning. Most families cope with their own problems,
even though they may sometimes be of quite severe intensity. However, accumulation or coincidence of stress in
a number of areas will predispose towards a breakdown of
family functioning irrespective of the initial and primary
stress (Rutter, 1977).

PROBLEMATIC RESPONSES TO THE FLASHPOINTS OF ADOLESCENT FAMILY INTERACTION

Any discussion of counselling the adolescent and his family
conducted in such a compressed form must necessarily be
schematic, but we believe that there is merit in efforts to
isolate and identify the general features involved. Thus,
building upon the interactive psycho-social model, we turn
briefly to examine reactions to the unresolved problems of
family and adolescent before turning to the task of the social
worker.
    The first issue that requires resolution is, when is a
problem a problem? We would suggest that if one of the
three possible participants, i.e. adolescent, parent or
'society' (as exemplified by the school, for instance), perceives that there is a difficulty then, if only at a highly subjective level, there is a problem to be resolved. Sometimes a resolution may be quickly achieved, e.g. when an
angry or anxious parent seeks advice but after careful
assessment the parent can be reassured and helped to deal
with his feelings towards his child in a more constructive
way. Equally an adolescent may be fearful of feelings or
relationships, or anxious about job or school. Again, competent assessment followed by reassurance can appropriately reduce the anxiety (Nuttall et al., 1977; Cerny, 1977).
The third participant is 'society' as represented by the
agencies of socialisation such as schools, police, social
service departments, educational welfare services etc.
(Robinson, 1978). Here the youngster is referred because
of some problem perceived by others. At the very least

this will require a more than superficial assessment and response from the social worker in conjunction with the adolescent and his parents.

Difficulties arising in any of the four constituent areas of functioning (emotional, social, economic and sexual) may be compounded by inappropriate responses from the family or the adolescent, or external social pressures may overwhelm the resources of the adolescent or his family.

Emotional areas

Some parents find difficulty in dealing with the adolescent's demands for independence. Others may dislike, or be disappointed in, the identity being evolved by their child because it does not match their own perceptions of, or aspirations for, him. The oscillating and inconsistent emotional demands of the adolescent may create in the parents severe anxiety or even hostility. Conversely some parents appear indifferent to the child's behaviour or emotional needs, or frankly reject him.

The adolescent commonly over-reacts to parental concern, misidentifying it as over-protectiveness or over-possessiveness. Yet confusingly he may interpret parental acceptance of his role and identity as lack of interest, or even rejection, particularly when he is rivalrous with his siblings. Perhaps the most disruptive response from the adolescent is one whereby, in his efforts to establish independence, he appears to emotionally reject his parents so that the parents find themselves 'tested' on every issue.

Socio-economic areas

A common parental response is to over-react to such symbols of adolescent style and status as dress, language, music or current fashions (e.g. the wearing of badges). This response may demonstrate a lack of sympathy with the adolescent generally, or a lack of understanding of the adolescent's need for peer acceptance and approval.

The social demands upon the adolescent can be considerable, especially if the norms and values of home and peer group clash. One frequent difficulty is that some youngsters fail to differentiate between what is the peer group's stated, or rather boasted, norm and what really occurs. Thus they believe assertions made by their peers about what they said to their parents and teachers, and then find that such behaviour creates a response from these adults with which they cannot deal.

Social responses to the adolescent are notoriously ambiguous. At one moment adolescents are treated as children

by the adult world, and often forcibly reminded of their
status; at the next, they are berated for their 'childish behaviour'. The responses of the mass media to the young
person must also appear very confusing – on the one hand,
as consumers, they are major targets for advertising cam-
paigns, on the other they are castigated as the disturbers
of the peace of respectable citizens (see Chapter two).

Sexual areas

Parents' response to the adolescent's sexuality is a frequent source of conflict that involves parent and young
person in very intense situations. The Freudian hypothesis of the oedipus complex is well known, and Kline (1972)
presents evidence which would support the existence of this
phenomenon in some measure. Rutter (1971) outlines what
to us is the most reasonable view, that in nuclear families
the potential for oedipal over-involvement exists. Where
it appears to be problematic is when a parent responds inappropriately to the child, becoming over-involved, or
places the young person in an incongruent role. Not infrequently, parents, in a genuine desire to protect their child
from potential exploitation and hurt, may express their concern in an over-anxious or hostile way and this becomes a
challenge for the adolescent to meet.

Adolescents' inappropriate response to their situation
can veer between a relative preoccupation with sex, with
accompanying anxiety as to how 'normal' they are in their
interest, or lack of interest, in it, to concern about their
sexual competence or attraction. One of the modern para-
doxes is that, amid the apparent plethora of open discussions and opportunities, young people may find it extremely
difficult to talk about such feelings with peers, or with anyone else. However, for the vast majority of adolescents,
conflicts and anxieties about sexual identity and experience
are relatively quickly resolved. Nevertheless it appears
that, for most, anxieties do occur, although these are
usually transient. However, there is certainly cause for
concern about the high incidence of teenage abortion
(31,000 in 1977 – 'Social Trends', 1979), illegitimacy, and
the serious shortage of counselling facilities for the young
people involved (Cheetham, 1977).

We now turn to the sexual and emotional problems of
parents and the repercussions of these problems upon their
children. It is not surprising that when a marriage breaks
down parents may sometimes be so preoccupied with their
own problems that they are unaware of those of their child-

ren. Parents may assume that if the ending of an unsatisfactory marriage or the acquisition of a new partner is a
good arrangement for them, it is also a good arrangement
for their children. This difficulty may be compounded by
the fact that many adolescents find great difficulty in talking
about their feelings, so that parents are encouraged to
think 'he isn't at all upset'.

Adolescents may, in fact, be extremely jealous when
parents form new sexual attachments or remarry. Many of
them would like to maintain contact with both parents, yet
a recent study showed that over half the children of separated parents lose contact with one parent within a few months
of the separation (Eckelaar et al., 1977). Similarly, the
step-parent faces great problems (see Maddox, 1975), for
which he is provided with little help. There is no role-
model readily available to him and he does not even enjoy
the benefits of the advice which is showered so freely upon
the 'natural' parent from all quarters.

FLIGHT OR FIGHT RESPONSES TO PROBLEMS IN YOUNG PEOPLE

What are the responses to these difficulties faced by adolescents and parents? Two broad, though not mutually exclusive, responses by families to intractable situations
appear to result in flight (neurotic, withdrawn reactions) or
fight (assertive, externalised behaviour). Again this is a
simple, schematic approach, but one helpful to our understanding of the components of a situation, and useful in that
much of the literature is presented within such implicit
categories (Eysenck, 1960; Freud, 1965).

Flight - neurotic and withdrawn behaviour

There is a qualitative difference between those families who
are close and mutually supportive and those who are over-
dependent, who, clinging together in a stress-producing
way, create an emotional atmosphere characterised by
tense anxiety and often suppressed aggression. On the one
hand their proximity poses a threat to each member, but
they also fear that a lessening of this over-closeness will
completely disrupt and fragment them. Frequently, the
prevailing anxiety is focused upon a particular family

member who appears to the outside world excessively shy,
withdrawn and fearful, often with complaints of minor physical indisposition (Pinckerton, 1974). Strong feelings,
especially anger, are often denied, which adds to the vicious circle of miscommunication and further suppression.
When children in such families come to adolescence, and
begin to make bids for independence, these moves will be
blocked by parents, as will their attempts to become involved in activities outside the family circle.

Fight – acting-out, externalised behaviour

The concept of acting-out originally came from the ego-
dynamic school of psychology, but has to a great extent
gained general acceptance. In essence the concept refers
to a person's response to social and emotional pressure,
which overwhelms his defence mechanisms, and results in
assertive/physical behaviour. This behaviour serves the
purpose of reducing emotional tension. The theory was
initially concerned with ideas of intra-psychic activity,
but it can easily be applied to external sources of stress,
such as a hostile social environment.

The acting-out response may occur in reaction to a variety of stimuli. For instance, a son may respond aggressively, sometimes even with physical aggression (Radin,
1967; Pritchard and Ward, 1974), to an over-involved
mother as he seeks to assert his independence and his masculinity. Conversely the rejecting parent may well evoke
counter-rejection, and instead of becoming predominantly
sad and depressed the youngster replies with externalised,
angry behaviour.

Parents who characteristically respond with acting-out,
externalised behaviour are likely to offer insufficient care
and control to their adolescent children, and may be anxious
to hand over the parenting function to social workers (see
Jordan, 1972, for a vivid account of his work with such
families).

To exemplify the flight/fight reactions we will explore a
problem often met by social workers who are involved with
families and adolescents, namely that of non-attendance at
school. The problem is often misunderstood and this can
lead to inappropriate referral or intervention (Pritchard,
1974).

Comparison of school phobia (flight) and truancy (fight)

It has been argued that viewing non-attendance at school
as 'abnormal' behaviour adopts an uncritical attitude to the
element of compulsion in the educational system, and col-
ludes with a middle-class view of normality (see Lang,
1974). However, the evidence emerging from retrospec-
tive studies of adult social and psychiatric 'casualties'
shows a strong association between poor school attendance
and subsequent adult breakdown (see, for example, Spinetta and Rigler, 1972, who looked at parents of abused children; McCulloch and Phillip, 1972, who studied adults involved in suicidal behaviour; and Garmezy and Streitman,
1974, who identified a number of school non-attenders who
subsequently developed psychoses). This is not to suggest that school non-attendance causes such problems, but
that it may be indicative of life-long stresses that first
become noticeable during childhood and adolescence. Consequently, we would urge the social worker to appreciate
the potential seriousness of school non-attendance, of
whatever type, rather than to uncritically, and perhaps
simplistically, accept that the justifiable criticisms which
may be made of our educational system negate any value
which the school may have for the child.
    School phobia has been differentiated from persistent
truancy by Hersov (1960), who noted the predominance of
anxiety, with restriction of behaviour, in the flight-respon-
sive school phobic, while the persistent truant is distinguished by his externalised, often aggressive behaviour.
Berg et al. (1969) succinctly define the characteristics of
the school phobic youngster as severe difficulty in attending
school, severe emotional upset, staying at home with the
parents' knowledge, and the absence of significant anti-
social behaviour. This is almost a complete reversal of
the truant (Turner, 1974).
    A particular difficulty in understanding the school phobic
is that when he is at school he is almost invariably well-
behaved and academically competent. This can confuse and
irritate teacher and social worker. The truant, however,
is rarely interested in school work and frequently experiences educational difficulties. He may also be involved in
disruption within the classroom when he does attend
school.
    Behaviour described as separation anxiety is often a
feature of school phobia (Eysenck and Rachman, 1964).

This may result in quite alarming distress for both parent and child at the prospect of being parted. Where boys are concerned there is often an over-involvement with the mother, and an apparently hostile response on the part of the father. Where a girl is involved, the relationship with her father may be inappropriately intense (Pritchard and Ward, 1974). Bleurer (1974) also noted a number of parents who were suffering from a psychiatric illness or breakdown (see also Berg et al., 1969) whose adolescent children failed to attend school and who were involved in a complex family interaction of separation anxiety and role reversal - the adolescent caring for the parent. In contrast, relationships between truants and their parents are characteristically indifferent or poor.

Hence we see that apparently similar behaviour (school non-attendance) can be promoted by differing ʻstresses and pressures, and therefore the tasks to be accomplished by the social worker are likely to be wide and varied. We now turn to explore some of these tasks.

THE TASKS OF THE SOCIAL WORKER

The tasks of the social worker can be broadly outlined under four headings:

Communication: Involving the adolescent and his family in meaningful communication with each other, with the worker and with other sources of help, and ensuring good inter-professional communication (see Chapter four). Perhaps we should also include under this heading facilitating the development of self-awareness and self-understanding as forms of communication with the self.

Care: By this we mean demonstrating concern for all involved (including members of one's own and other agencies!) and, where appropriate, offering a sustaining and ameliorative relationship.

Change: Intervention in any situation implies change. The worker's role may range from mediating in a fraught family interaction to ensuring that all available resources are mobilised for the family.

Control: The worker must sometimes take on a controlling function in situations where, if no halt is called, custodial care is likely to result with the associated increasingly poor outcome (Farrington, 1978; Hoghughi, 1978b).

Such a range of tasks demands a highly flexible response

from the worker, involving him in a series of different roles ranging from therapist and adviser to advocate, co-ordinator and broker (see Baker, 1976, for a list of linking and overlapping roles). The tasks are geared to the overall aim of solving or alleviating the problem, or, where neither is possible, ensuring that the problem has been thoroughly explored and that those concerned have a realistic understanding of its nature. An example of the achievement of this last aim concerns an adolescent boy, who was labelled by his school as being 'severely emotionally disturbed' and 'beyond control' on the basis of a few minutes' infantile, unrestrained behaviour, and in the knowledge that the boy's father had a history of chronic mental illness. The social worker was unable to persuade the family that she might be of help to them, but was able to assemble the evidence, reassess the situation, and point out to the school the inappropriate nature of the label that was being attached to the boy.

Many adolescent problems involve both adolescent and parents, so that the social worker is immediately faced with the problems of how to present herself as helpful to possibly contending parties. Should she concentrate upon working with the adolescent, with the parents, or with both – in which case should she see them separately or use joint interviewing techniques?

Decisions about who is to be worked with may be taken because the social worker finds it easier to work with certain groups of clients. Many young social workers find it easy to empathise and identify with adolescents, as they have so recently gone through this developmental stage themselves. They may find it more difficult to understand the point of view of parents and to relate to them. Parents may compound this difficulty by challenging the credibility of the young social worker, and by asking searching questions about her experience and whether she has children of her own. Conversely many older social workers feel more comfortable working with parents, and find difficulty in communicating with adolescents or in breaking through the adolescent's stereotyped image of the middle aged. Again, parents may compound this problem by presenting the social worker to the adolescent as an adult authority figure who has come to support the parents' point of view.

While it is important for the worker to be aware of her own particular skills and preferred way of working, these should not be the primary criteria upon which decisions

about methods of intervention are based.   The possibility
of colluding with the view of the situation presented by adolescent or parents, and the consequent likelihood of failing
to effect an improvement in the situation, are obvious.   An
example of this process occurring was seen in the case of a
15-year-old girl, who had been identified by the general
practitioner as 'driving her mother to the edge of a nervous
breakdown'.   The first social worker involved in the case
identified very strongly with the mother, and repeatedly
lectured the girl about her behaviour – to no apparent
effect.   The second social worker, who became involved at
the point of the girl running away from home, insisted upon
seeing mother and daughter together.   She pointed out that
both mother and daughter were contributing to the unhappy
relationship which existed between them, and that the
mother was almost 'imposing' behaviour upon her daughter
by suggesting that she would behave in certain, unacceptable ways.   She helped the girl to talk to her mother about
her grief at the abortion which she (the girl) had undergone
some months earlier – a subject which had not previously
been discussed between them.   The relationship between
mother and daughter improved to the point at which they
were able to agree that the girl would remain at home rather
than go into care, which had been the original suggestion,
but that the social worker would help her to find other
accommodation when the girl left school.

It seems to us that much successful intervention in adolescent problems, particularly where the problem is located
in relationships within the family, depends upon the social
worker facilitating a process of bargaining between adolescent and parents.   The social worker may also form an important modelling role for parents and for adolescent (e.g.
by insisting upon listening carefully to the views of all concerned).   Decisions as to whether to work separately with
parents and adolescents might, however, hinge upon whether
the aim is to reintegrate the adolescent into the family or to
aid a 'developmental separation' (for example, in the case
quoted above, the social worker would probably choose to
work separately with the mother and the girl when plans
were being made for the girl to leave home).

THE DEVELOPMENT OF A COMMITTED INTERVENTION RELATIONSHIP

The most significant factor to emerge from research into all forms of psycho-social intervention in the last decade is the importance of the relationship context in which the intervention takes place. Rogers (1971) clearly demonstrates this within his 'client-centred therapy'. From the fields of psychiatry (Clare, 1976) and behavioural psychology (Shepherd and Richardson, 1979) there are also frequent reports of the enhancement of treatment processes when these are based upon an effective relationship.
Smale (1977) points out that the well-established concept of the self-fulfilling prophecy is applicable to social work.
He shows that a positive relationship aids the client in changing his behaviour, or in coping with his problems, and that a negative approach can actually be damaging to the client.

The components of a sustaining and change-enabling relationship are what Rogers (1971) calls congruence (that is a genuine and honest response to the client), unconditional regard (affirmation of an individual's worth irrespective of his situation), and empathetic understanding (an ability not only to understand the client, but to demonstrate that understanding to him). It is also possible to distinguish stages in the relationship between worker and client and these are described by Butrym (1976) and Baker (1976) in a way which we have found helpful for clarifying the interaction.

The beginning phase

(a) Pre-contact: The majority of clients who come to social work agencies are referred by a third party. It is important therefore that social workers ensure that the function of their agency and its way of working are well known to those organisations that are likely to refer adolescents (e.g. schools, general practitioners), and that information about the agency is widely disseminated through the community at large. As Rees (1978) says 'Those who influence others in contacting a social worker are potential image makers' and Burck (1978), in a research project on referrals to a child guidance clinic, showed how little those who were responsible for initiating referrals under-

stood about the working of the service. Hence, stereotypes
of the professional social work role may be highly mislead-
ing, yet potentially powerful. It is our impression that
social workers are popularly seen as performing only a
social control function with respect to adolescents so that,
unless we are content with this stereotype of the social work
role, we must take steps to amend it.

(b) Initial contact: We need to be aware of what significance contact with the agency may have for the client.
Rees (1978), in a study of clients of a local authority
department and a voluntary agency, found that half his
sample said that they had experienced feelings of shame at
being referred to a social worker. Impressions gained by
adolescents and their parents through telephone calls to the
agency, contacts with receptionists (Hall, 1974), and duty
officers, or by letter (Timms, 1972) may be extremely influential in setting the tone of the contact, for at this stage
they are likely to be particularly sensitive to the badly
worded letter or message. The worker must quickly develop a rapport with the adolescent and his parents which
will enable them to be as frank as possible in discussing
their problem. If they have not referred themselves, they
may be very puzzled about the role of the agency and of the
worker, so that the worker should be prepared to take the
initiative in talking about what he and the agency may be
able to offer.

The middle phase

This is the time at which the major work of tackling the
problem is undertaken. As Butrym (1976) points out,
ambivalence is a common feature of this stage. The task
may prove more difficult than was originally envisaged by
adolescent, parent or worker and there may be considerable uncertainty on the part of those involved as to whether
they are prepared to face the implications of change. This
may be particularly the case where the adolescent was originally identified as 'the problem' but when further assessment suggests that it is in fact a family problem.

The end phase – termination

The ending of cases, or of the social worker's contact with a client, needs to be prepared well in advance. Feelings of loss may emerge at this time, especially where there has been a warm and valued relationship, and there is a danger that client or worker may deal with these feelings by means of denial or anger. An important example of this is when a social worker terminates his contract with an adolescent in care. Much thought needs to be given as to how this will be done, who is to be the new worker, and how she will be introduced to the adolescent. Although we appreciate that agencies often face considerable problems in terms of staffing, it has to be realised that from the adolescent's perspective a badly managed change of worker demonstrates only abandonment and lack of caring.

LONG- OR SHORT-TERM INTERVENTION?

Evidence from the USA (see, for example, Fowler, 1967), suggests that few clients are motivated to continue in long-term treatment. Kogan (1957), in a follow-up study of clients who had withdrawn from treatment, found that the majority of them claimed that the problems for which they had requested help had, at least partially, been resolved. Reid and Shyne (1969), in a carefully structured study of families with inter-personal problems, showed that clients receiving short-term focused casework help achieved significantly more positive change than those receiving long-term open-ended help.

It seems to us that there are many arguments in favour of aiming for short-term intervention, where appropriate, when working with adolescents and their parents. There is very much less risk of encouraging dependency and of setting unrealistic goals. Worker, adolescent and parents are likely to be able to maintain their level of motivation and to work harder, and in a more focused way, knowing that there is a limited time within which they can achieve their goals. Where a crisis exists, motivation is often high, and short-term, intensive intervention is, therefore, much more likely to be effective. For example, parents may be prepared to consider that problems exist around the time of a suicide gesture made by their teenage daughter, but a few days later may rationalise the happening and insist that all is well.

Obviously there are situations (such as that outlined in the case study at the end of the chapter) in which short-term intervention would be of little value. In some cases the social worker has a statutory duty to maintain contact with an adolescent over a long period, as, for instance, when a probation order or a supervision order has been made. If long-term intervention is to be successful, then it is important that focus and motivation are not lost. There is a need for periodic reassessments with the adolescent and his family of what is being achieved and what new goals should be worked towards (see Parker, 1971).

PLANNING WITH THE CLIENT

Planning with the client has received increasing emphasis in recent social work literature. The psycho-social model of casework (Hollis, 1974) emphasised much more the importance of the worker's understanding of the situation, but consumer studies have shown how unacceptable this traditional approach can be. Mayer and Timms (1970), for example, point out the frustration and anger felt by some clients when the purpose of their contact with the social worker was not clarified or agreed upon between them. Robinson (1978), writing as the father of a handicapped child and consequently as a consumer of professional welfare services, argues powerfully that professional-client 'encounters' should be structured to give the client 'a more equal status in the encounter and to improve the flow of communication in both directions'.

Hutten (1977) and Reid and Epstein (1972) suggest that making an explicit contract with the client will help both worker and client move towards the achievement of shared goals. When working with the adolescent and his parents, it is obviously essential that the purpose of the intervention should be agreed upon and clearly understood by everyone concerned, for, as we have seen, adolescent and parent may have conflicting expectations of the worker, and each may be attempting to enlist the support of the worker on his behalf. A written contract will be useful in some circumstances, but in other circumstances, a firm verbal agreement will be adequate. Sometimes a contract will have to be provisional and be revised from interview to interview. In addition to goals, the contract should specify the length of the intervention, the number of meetings between worker

and client, how these will be arranged, and the tasks
which client and worker will be expected to carry out.
    The setting of specific tasks ('what the client is to do to
alleviate his problem') (Reid and Epstein, 1972) has recently become increasingly popular with social workers. The
term 'task' is of course in common use in family therapy
(sometimes in the form of 'homework'), and is linked to
recent emphases in the field of learning theory that 'people
learn best by doing'. Further developments of the task-
centred approach (Reid and Epstein, 1977) have extended
the concept of task to include 'tasks carried out by the
worker', and 'thinking tasks'. This last classification
fits in well with the value placed upon reflection by such
writers as Hollis (1974), Nursten (1974) and Hutten (1977).
An interesting development of the crisis-intervention model
has been made by Golan (1978), who shows how a task-
centred approach can be used in a rapidly changing situation. She gives a particularly valuable example of its use
when working with an adolescent and his family.
    Certainly a task-centred approach is well fitted in many
ways to work with adolescents. Reciprocal tasks can be
agreed upon (e.g. for.the adolescent: 'John is to come in
by 11 p.m. every evening during the next two weeks, and
for the parents: 'During this same period Mr and Mrs Smith
will not criticise John's friends or his appearance'). Such
a strategy fits in well with the bargaining approach to family
problems which we have already outlined. Moreover, the
approach is concrete, specific and short-term, all of which
are factors which may recommend it to the adolescents.

COUNSELLING ROLES - ALTERNATIVE STRATEGIES

We would like to put forward an eclectic approach, which is
based upon, or has been influenced by, a number of writers
from the social and behavioural sciences. We do not feel
that any one model is adequate to cover intervention in the
range of adolescent situations with which social workers
have to deal.
    The first group of models to which we will refer includes
the psycho-dynamic approach as outlined by Hollis (1974),
Nursten (1974) and Rogers (1971) with its emphasis upon the
value of a warm, empathetic relationship, and the importance of support, ventilation and reflection. It also includes the crisis-intervention model as developed by

Rapoport (1970) and Golan (1978), which underlines the
importance of developmental transitions, and links this concept with that of age-specific tasks which must be carried
out by parent and adolescent. We also draw upon a second
group of models from the literature on family therapy, see
for example Satir (1967) and Walrond-Skinner (1976).
Family therapy with its emphasis upon the patterns of
family communication and transactions offers a potentially
valuable method of intervention when working with adolescents and their families. Third, the writings of the various systems theorists (e.g. Pincus and Minahan, 1973;
Goldstein, 1973) have encouraged us to consider the whole
range of systems which impinge upon the adolescent and
his family, and confirmed the value of indirect work carried out on behalf of the client. Finally the modern behav-
iourists have strongly directed our thinking into specific
forms of intervention techniques that are appropriate for
particular pieces of behaviour that either require diminution or expansion (see Jehu et al., 1972; Lazarus, 1976).

THE TASK OF THE SOCIAL WORKER - AN EXAMPLE

The following case example is presented as an attempt to
illustrate in an integrated way some of the themes which
emerge when considering the intervention of the social
worker. Demands of space and ease of presentation have
required a major compression of the stages of development
of the situation, so that it now appears more schematically
coherent than it did in practice. We mention this because
case examples in text books often appear so sequentially
logical that the confusion, anxiety, and indecision of the
worker, which are common to almost every complex situation, are lost, and the reader can easily become demora-
lised by the standards of perfection which appear to be
offered.

At an area case conference, it was agreed that Mr Smith,
a social worker attached to a child guidance clinic,
should act as the key worker in the case of Mary Adams,
a 13-year-old girl who had not attended school for almost
a year. The Adams family was well known to a number
of social work agencies, schools, general practitioner
and the police, but no agency had succeeded in establishing a working relationship with them. It was hoped that
Mr Smith would be able to devote rather more time to the

case than had been possible for the social workers previously involved, and that he would give particular attention to facilitating liaison between the many agencies
concerned.

Mr Smith was new to the area and to the agency. He
was, consequently, very anxious to succeed, but deeply
concerned that he might fail, especially in view of the
complex nature of the case and the obvious pessimism of
those who knew the family.

Mary, since the age of 3, because of polio, had suffered from a severely deformed leg. She wore an iron
caliper, and there was some shortening of her right arm.
Her father, aged 36 years, an ex-semi-professional
sportsman, had been involved in a serious industrial
accident 5 years previously and this had exacerbated his
tendency to heavy drinking. He had a reputation of
being a local 'tough', well known to the police because of
a number of physical assaults. Mary's mother, aged 31
years, had been involved with the police because of shop-
lifting 4 years previously and was known to the GP because of 'nerves'. She had recently been very abusive
to Mary's teachers, accusing them of 'picking on Mary
because of her leg', and threatening to get Mr Adams to
'deal with them'. Following this Michael, aged 11 years,
and John, 9 years, had begun to attend school only spor-
adically, apparently in response to what the family regarded as the unsympathetic handling of Mary's school
difficulties. An ultimatum had been given that unless
Mary recommenced school the parents would be prosecu-
ted and that there would be a very real possibility that
Mary might be taken into the care of the local authority.

There are a number of points which we can note prior to
the worker's first visit to the family. First, Mary's non-
attendance at school appears to have started around the
time of her transfer from primary to secondary school. It
will be important, therefore, for the social worker to examine in some detail the circumstances surrounding the
transfer, the attitude of Mary and her parents to the school,
and the attitude of the school staff towards Mary and her
parents.

Second, Mary has arrived at an age at which she is
likely to be preoccupied with the question of her own personal and sexual identity. The fact that she has a noticeable physical handicap may complicate this process, and
may make it difficult for her to form a clear self-concept.

During adolescence many young people are particularly
conscious of their physical appearance, and they may be
cast into the depths of despair because of a slight deviation
from an assumed ideal physical appearance. For Mary the
discrepancy between the ideal and the reality may be all the
more difficult to bear and may cause her to have fundamental doubts about her personal and sexual attractiveness.

Third, the Adams family are facing a complex of interacting problems in the areas of finance, health, and social
relations, and are responding to these problems with mixed
fight/flight reactions. The fact that their responses are
so unpredictable is likely to make the social worker's first
approach a difficult one.

On the first visit to the home, which had been preceded
by a letter of appointment, Mr Smith was verbally abused
by Mrs Adams from an upstairs window, threatened with
the dog, warned of the violence of Mr Adams, and finally
had water thrown on him. He retreated feeling angry,
confused and damp! On reflection he decided to write
again at once because, as he stated in his letter, while
the family were undoubtedly angry, they couldn't be
angry with Mr Smith, whom they had never met. He emphasised that he would like to hear the family's side of
the story, and arranged to call again in a few days' time.

On this occasion Mr Smith was received grudgingly by
Mrs Adams and kept on the doorstep for half an hour,
while she availed herself of the opportunity of giving him
'a piece of her mind' and of passing on her defiance of
'the council and all the others'. Mr Smith listened and
recognised her real anguish about the threat of the re-
moval of Mary, and her sense of despair, anger and confusion as to what was going on around her. Mrs Adams
finally agreed that Mr Smith should come into the house.
He was able to express some genuinely felt sympathy for
her plight, but gently and firmly pointed out the parameters of his responsibility in an effort to deal with the
implicit 'authority' situation. Mrs Adams expressed
understandable irritation about being 'threatened', but
begrudgingly agreed to further contact. She refused,
however, to agree to the worker's suggestion that her
husband should be present on the next occasion, saying
'He'd kill you. He gets so mad'.

During the initial contact with Mrs Adams the worker
focuses on building a relationship, and attempting to reduce
her level of anxiety. In many such situations so much

pressure has been exerted upon the family that they have become completely paralysed by anxiety.   The worker will then have to go at a slower pace in order to establish a rapport with the family.   In addition he may have to persuade any other agencies involved of the effectiveness of such an approach.   There are situations, of course, in which the social worker needs to make a family more anxious; however, our experience suggests that these situations do not occur as frequently as is commonly supposed, and that what passes for indifference on the part of a family is often the paralysing anxiety to which we refer above.

Major strides were made during the next two visits, although Mrs Adams still refused to agree that her husband should be present.   She took the opportunity to express considerable anger and fear of the future and also began to talk about her own sense of guilt concerning Mary's handicap.   An orthopaedic surgeon had bluntly criticised her for not having Mary vaccinated.   During these visits the boys remained upstairs and Mary was absent, visiting her paternal grandmother.

It was agreed that Mr Smith would attempt to arrange an adjournment of the court hearing (this involved frantic activity on the part of himself and his senior in order to gain the agreement of the educational services).   It was agreed that the boys would return to school, and that Mr Smith would accompany them on the first occasion as they were very apprehensive about returning after a long period of absence.   In fact the school proved very sympathetic to the needs of the boys, both of whom settled down quickly, and the boys admitted that they were pleased 'to get out of our Mary's way'.

At this stage in the intervention Mrs Adams is still displaying what Seligman (1975) calls 'learned helplessness'. The social worker concentrates upon providing opportunities for her to talk about her feelings (particularly important in view of her social isolation), and upon carrying out tasks himself which will both help to remove pressure from the family and demonstrate that the situation can be improved by means of positive action.

Over the next month all appeared to be going well especially in the creation of a relationship with Mrs Adams, who seemed rather more relaxed now that she could talk about some of her anxieties.   Mrs Adams felt herself to be in a very isolated position.   She had been the only child of a single mother, who had given her very little

affection.   She had left home at 16 and met and married
Mr Adams when she was 18.

At this point the worker's assessment centred largely
upon an over-protective mother made guilty by the damage
to a much wanted daughter, from whom she had hoped to
gain some of the affection of which she herself had been
deprived.   However, the social situation made matters
worse.   Mrs Adams was shunned by her neighbours because of her husband's reputation, and she was resented
by her mother-in-law, who had disapproved of the marriage.   Moreover, the family was chronically short of
money because of Mr Adams's intermittent unemployment.

Communication between the parents was difficult.   Mr
Adams's behaviour was totally unpredictable.   At times
he appeared to rely completely upon his wife, at other
times he beat her.   He dealt with external problems by
means of threats or actual violence (e.g. he had spent
one month in prison for severely beating a neighbour who
had made complaints about Mary).

Now we become more aware of the complex of problems
facing the family in social, economic and sexual spheres.
Mrs Adams is likely to be threatened by Mary's arrival at
adolescence, because for Mrs Adams motherhood represents an ideal role which she may be loathe to abandon, and
the marital relationship offers little consistent support for
her in facing the necessary changes in 'letting Mary go'.

Mrs Adams was genuinely distressed by the bullying to
which Mary had been subjected at school and by the fact
that Mary was rejected by her peers.   Undoubtedly the
school was less than sympathetic to Mary, despite statements by the headmaster that the staff had always tried to
'meet the Adams halfway'.   The school, which was in a
deprived area, had many other problems with which they
had to deal besides those of Mary.   The headmaster was
concerned lest concessions to Mary might be thought of as
a precedent and taken advantage of by other parents and
children.

Although the worker has yet to meet Mary, he must already be considering the desirability of her transfer to a
school in which the staff would be more sympathetic to her
needs, and in which good pastoral care would be available.

Mr Smith felt that Mrs Adams now had sufficient trust in
him to allow him to meet Mary and Mr Adams - although it
must be admitted that by now he was quite apprehensive
about meeting the latter, as Mrs Adams had continued to

impress him with stories of her husband's uncontrollable
rage and violence together with his dislike of all social
workers.

At the first meeting with Mr Adams there was a tense
20 minutes, during which Mr Adams lived up to his label
of being a 'tough' by his attitude and gestures, and then
by verbally challenging the worker, who felt his masculinity under threat. This was partly because Mr Smith
did not want to appear weak in front of Mrs Adams, and
also because of the cultural pressures upon him to stand
up to the challenge. With difficulty he set aside the
threat and showed that he was not competing for control
of the interview, but sought only to determine Mr Adams's
view of the situation.

There was a grave danger that if contact with Mr Adams
had been delayed much longer it might have becom impossible because of his resentment at the worker's relationship
with Mrs Adams, and that this might have led to a further
deterioration in the family situation. We can see already
some pressure upon the worker to respond to Mrs Adams's
rather idealised view of him.

Mr Adams now relaxed and expressed some of his feelings
about being 'got at by everybody - if I don't stand up to
them I'm a nobody'. It began to emerge that not only did
Mr Adams feel compelled to maintain his image, but that
Mrs Adams frequently used his reputation in a defensive
and manipulative way. Towards the end of the session
Mr Adams and the worker were beginning to create a
rapport, and then Mary arrived home from her grandmother's.

The whole situation changed. Mary ignored Mr Smith.
She abused her parents for their 'betrayal' of her, and
made a series of conflicting demands, which quickly reduced the parents to a state of anxious, guilt-ridden
impotence.

Mr Smith was aware of his negative feelings towards
this child, who resolutely rejected all his efforts to make
contact with her. Rational communication was impossible, and he realised that his previous assessment was
in many ways seriously at variance with reality. For
the first time in his contact with the family he decided
that it was essential that he gain firm control of the interview. Quietly, but with determination, he said to Mary
that he realised that she did not want to speak to him at
the moment, and that she should wait in the kitchen until

her parents had finished talking to him. Mr Smith was
very relieved when Mary did in fact storm out to the
kitchen, swearing and shouting. Her parents, despite
their obvious surprise that she had done what was asked
of her, and their obvious discomfort in the situation,
stayed put. Mr Smith reinforced her father's decision
to 'leave her in peace'. After some desultory moments,
both parents began to complain about Mary's assertiveness, their inability to control her, and their resentment
at being blamed by everyone for her behaviour. They
made a direct appeal to the worker to help them, 'because
we don't know what to do next'. The worker quickly
arranged another meeting in the near future.

We see here the worker 'modelling' an appropriate way to
deal with Mary, and refusing to become drawn into the
family interaction. He is careful, however, not to over-
respond to the family's appeal to help them. Jordan points
out (1972) the danger of the social worker adopting a quasi-
parental role, and the importance of not colluding with
parents' view of their own ineptitude.

The situation was not fully resolved for another 18
months. During this period Mary very happily settled
into a special boarding school for 'delicate' children.
Mr Smith had to completely redefine the problem, not
only in relation to the other agencies involved, but also
in relation to his own assessment and his preconceptions
about a sad, crippled child. This last factor was of
crucial importance in understanding everyone's response
to the family. No one, least of all her parents, could
admit to themselves that she was a 'problem' in her own
right, as all sought to 'excuse' her dominating, bullying
behaviour for which, they felt, she could not be held responsible, because of her handicap.

The course of intervention went as follows - reapprais-
ing the situation the worker recognised that each member
of the family had emotional and social needs that were not
being met. A colleague was enlisted to work primarily
with Mary, as it was felt that she needed a great deal of
help in her own right. She eventually admitted to her
social worker that she 'enjoyed' the power she exercised
at home as 'it serves them right'. The two boys were
relieved of their burden of being made to feel sorry for
Mary, and in some way responsible for her handicap.
They were no longer prohibited from retaliating when
Mary attacked them and thus no longer reinforced her

undesirable behaviour. The fact that Mr and Mrs Adams
were becoming less preoccupied with Mary meant that
they had more time for the two boys, and Mr Adams in
particular spent more time with them and less time away
from home after the value the boys placed upon his company had been pointed out to him. The positive feelings
in the family were reinforced, and although there were
many difficulties, over the months the violence in the
family decreased.

Perhaps the greatest problem was how to help Mary to
come to terms with her disability and to realise her un-
doubted potential. She was of good intelligence, and her
handicap interfered only marginally with her ability to
live a 'normal' life. Yet much of Mary's life had been
taken up with self-destructive behaviour.

After a number of family conferences, including both
workers, it was decided that it would not be in the interests of either Mary or her family for her to return to her
previous school (this decision had subsequently to be
fought through the case conference because the headmaster believed that it reflected adversely upon his school).
It was recognised that Mary needed some success, and
that she should not have to maintain her 'bad' image. It
was also felt that it would be difficult for Mary to change
her behaviour in such a fundamental way if she remained
at home. Consequently the decision was made to place
her in a boarding school where she would be able to
achieve scholastically, and where she would be encouraged to build up a different pattern of behaviour. Financial help was obtained to enable her parents to visit fort-
nightly. Mary returned home every half term and, in her
last year at school, every weekend. Her parents found
great support in belonging to a parents group at the
school of which they eventually became key members.

Finally let us summarise some of the work carried out in
this case. First, the worker redefined the problem for the
various agencies concerned, so that they were able to
appreciate the total family situation and actively support
efforts on behalf of the family. This involved the worker
in advocacy, intercession and liaison roles. It also provided him with an opportunity to ventilate some of the frustration and despair which he often felt when working with
this family, and to support workers in other agencies when
they had to face similar feelings.

Second, the worker established a relationship with both

parents and he recognised their needs. He helped the parents to come to terms with the 'loss' of their child once it became obvious that Mary would be able to support herself in the outside world. Financial help and co-operation from the housing department were also important factors during the early months of the contact.

Third, Mr Smith and his colleague provided models for the parents in their response to Mary and helped them to cope with her in a much more confident manner. The second worker offered Mary a confidential relationship in her own right, and as the second worker was senior to Mr Smith she particularly enjoyed the reflected status.

Fourth, the worker's primary aim of reintegration was achieved by facing his own and others' guilt in appearing to 'punish' Mary when it was decided that a 'developmental separation' would be the interim aim before reintegration into the family was possible.

Fifth, because of good support and supervision within the team, the worker was able to be honest enough about his competitive feelings in regard to Mr Adams and later to his senior colleague's success with the intransigent Mary.

Finally, the workers were able to bring about more open communication within the family, and hope that things could change. This resulted in recognition of the way in which inflexible roles had been allocated within the family, and of the need for family members to be allowed to develop as individuals in their own right. The boys in particular showed tremendous gains in the educational field and in their social life.

SUMMARY

In reflecting on this chapter, and on the case study, we would wish to emphasise that the problems of the adolescent should be considered within the context in which they occur. Many problems arise in the family, and we have argued that parents are often caught up in their own mid-life crisis, and that, where this is so, attention needs to be focused upon their predicament.

We have identified some crucial issues – the importance of developing a positive relationship; attempting an imaginative understanding of the situation of both parent and adolescent; and the value of planning with them. Finally, we would like to stress the importance of 'focus' (concentrating

upon a problem or a segment of a problem where it is likely
that change can be effected) and 'structure' (creating a
framework which is agreed upon by worker, adolescent and
parent, and which will assist them in working effectively
towards a resolution of the problem).

Chapter six

Groupwork with adolescents

Andrew Kerslake

/The previous chapter explored some of the issues which
arise between parents and adolescents, and the implications
for the social worker who has the task of counselling adolescents and their families. This chapter uses a similar
approach of looking at 'normal' adolescent development and
concerns, but its focus is the adolescent and his peer group.
The chapter discusses some of the factors which should be
considered when working with adolescent groups. It also
explores some of the settings in which this groupwork may
occur, but its primary focus is groupwork undertaken by
fieldworkers.7

THE INFLUENCE OF THE PEER GROUP

That the peer group plays an important part in our life is a
statement with which most people would agree, but the vast
amount of written material on human development suggests
that it assumes an even greater importance during the particular developmental stage of adolescence. The adolescents' peers offer a reference group when greater independence from the family is being sought, and provide an alternative source of values.
    The popular image, which is given a great deal of cre-
dence by the media, sees the adolescent peer group primarily as a threat, which can range from petty vandalism to gang
warfare, and even some social workers view working with
adolescents as, at best, 'difficult' (see Chapter nine). To
understand the peer group, and the extent to which it should
influence decisions about social work practice, particularly
within the 'formed group', calls for a review of the research

material relating to adolescence, and this is attempted below.

Conger (1973) and others observe that individual friendships can be just as important to the adolescent as group influence, and that the nature of adolescent friendships, and the need to conform to the peer group, change significantly with age. In examining the relationship between the adolescent and his parents they find the assumption that parental and peer group influences are mutually exclusive is not well founded (see Chapter two). The amount of parental influence varies according to the age of the child and to the subject being influenced, and, while the peer group is likely to have a greater effect on styles of clothing and music, the parents usually maintain influence over the adolescent's moral and social values.

This view is supported by Davies who, whilst emphasising the inter-relationship of parental and peer influence, also stresses the importance of the peer group for the adolescent:

Contemporaries, then, are not the only, or even the predominant influence as to what adolescents do or think. Their views are felt in only limited and passing areas of the adolescent's life. And yet within the areas they affect, their influence is significant and obvious because for the adolescent these areas are important. That is why 'helpers' like teachers and social workers who ignore or actively reject the group to which the adolescent belongs (even if they feel sympathetic to him individually) are liable themselves to be rejected (Davies, 1975, p. 716).

Clearly some parent-adolescent relationships experience what has been termed the 'generation gap' more than others. This is reflected in the research literature, so that some writers (Coleman, 1961; Friedenburg, 1969) see the development of an alienated youth culture, whilst others (e.g. Lesser and Kandel, 1969; Offer and Offer, 1969; Bandura, 1970) find that adolescents do not, on the whole, go through a period of extended rebellion and hostility to parents. One reason why these differences occur has been put forward by Larson (1975) who sees the quality of the relationships in the home as an important determinant when examining the relative attractiveness of the peer group. In what he calls the 'parent-adolescent affect' he sees those who have the most rewarding and positive parental relationships as being those most influenced by their parents. Conversely those with poor relationships show a greater need to differentiate between the influence of their parents and their best friends. Larson found that parental influence decreased with age, and that although there was little correlation during early adolescence between the quality of the parent-child relationship and parental influence, the 'parental-adolescent affect' assumed greater importance in determining parental influence during adolescence. As Conger states in commenting on Larson's work:

> In short if a parent thinks that because he can influence his children at the beginning of adolescence without concerning himself with the quality of the relationship with his children and his contribution to it, and that he will continue to be able to do so in middle and later adolescence, then he may be making a big mistake (Conger, 1975, p. 276).

Therefore the significant factor in some adolescent-parent difficulties lies at the interaction of the moral and social values (taken from the parents) and the cultural and life-style orientation (largely determined by the peer group). Although a generalisation, problems often seem to arise when either the parents fail to achieve a relationship of trust, or where the domineering parent fails to allow the adolescent to be integrated into the peer group. Parents in this situation often perceive staying out late, going to parties, or bizarre forms of dress as an attack on their values and translate them into various forms of potential immorality or outright rebellion, rather than accepting them as a cultural and stylistic stance by the adolescent. This adoption of poses or postures by the peer group is illustrated, for example, by Marsh (1978) on football hooligans. Here the 'ritual' of the fight, the 'squaring-up' and 'not losing face' display of aggression, assumes a far greater importance than actual physical contact, which rarely occurs despite the image conveyed by the mass media.

The idea that the peer group is a single, identifiable body which exists throughout adolescence would also seem to be a mistaken view. Various authors (see Dunphy, 1963) have identified varying sizes of groups during adolescence, from individual friendships, through cliques or small groups, to large crowds or gangs. The latter category normally acts as a reservoir for changing friendship patterns or allegiances from which the smaller groupings can be drawn. Even here parents can still exert a large amount of influence by physical factors, such as where the home is situated, which school the adolescent attends, by 'chaperonage'

as a means of avoiding delinquency amongst the peer group
(Wilson, 1974), or even by direct disapproval. In Coleman's (1961) study, for instance, 70 per cent of the adolescents questioned said that they would not join a club if their
parents disapproved.

These changes in the size and nature of adolescent friendship groupings also relate to the concept of differing stages
within adolescent development. Blos (1962) saw this development as alternating between pushes towards an adult
identity and regression towards childhood. Dunphy (1963)
offers a chart (see Figure 6.1) which depicts these stages
of development within the peer group.

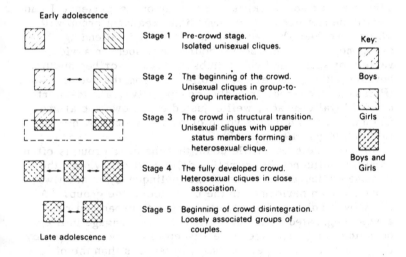

FIGURE 6.1 Stages of group development during adolescence (from Dunphy, 1963)

Figure 6.1 shows that during adolescence the peer group
develops from clearly defined uni-sexual groupings (the
sneer from the 10-year-old boy of 'Who wants to play with
girls?') into a secondary phase where some heterosexual
interaction takes place, but only with the support of the
whole group, and even then this is marked by a high degree
of approach/avoidance behaviour and a public face of ambivalence. The third phase is initiated when the higher
status, more mature group members begin to form heterosexual couples, and this process gradually permeates

throughout the group by the time the fourth and fifth stages
are reached. Although no age boundaries are ascribed to
the various stages, as wide variation from individual to individual occurs, the influence of age not only relates to the
sex and type of friendships formed, but also their permanency.

A central focus for the social worker, if not for the whole
community, is the potential of the peer group to be involved
in delinquent acts, especially amongst those whose material
and physical environments are limited, where few strong
internalised prohibitions exist, and where such behaviour
offers status within the group. This is not to infer that
members of delinquent groups show a low level of social
adjustment or social skills. From my own experience I can
recall one member of an intermediate treatment group with
which I worked who had genuine difficulty in attending
group meetings as his social hours were spent in a wide
variety of sports and youth clubs. Mays describes another
boy who although a persistent offender from the age of 9 was:
'Pleasant-mannered, friendly, co-operative, a true-sports-
man, a loyal comrade, well adjusted to his own social group
and milieu, active in his youth club, and adored by his
mother' (Mays, 1954, p. 68).

Whilst there seems little doubt that the peer group is often
an active influence in promoting delinquent behaviour, there
is some evidence which shows that delinquency is not always
a phenomenon performed in the presence of the group. A
study by Hindlelang (1976), covering both urban and rural
areas, suggested that whilst offenders who engage in illegal
behaviour in groups are more susceptible to being caught by
the police, a far larger number of offenders than the official
statistics suggest are likely to commit delinquent acts alone.
Some offences, such as those involving drugs, tended to be
group phenomena, but a higher number of theft and property
damage charges were, according to Hindlelang, committed
either always or usually alone. Despite this, the majority
of evidence still points to juvenile delinquency being a group
phenomenon. A study by Shapland (1978) shows that group
offences account for the majority of delinquent activities,
although, as might be expected, there are variations according to the type of offence committed, and in the size of the
group involved.

THE ADOLESCENT GROUP AND SOCIAL WORK

From the research discussed above, it can be seen that various qualifications should be considered when talking about the adolescent peer group; its influence is often limited, its composition can vary according to age, and its appearance of solidarity challenged. Yet it is important to remember that the discussion so far has been a normative one, for many of the adolescents that social workers meet are likely to experience a greater degree of peer group influence than the normative model suggests.

This provides one rationale for social workers to undertake groupwork with adolescents, as for the social worker the adoption of any method should be founded on the problem or issue to be solved. However, the worker's own preference is also an important consideration. Whilst that preference might be for neighbourhood work (see Chapter seven), limitations on time, and the duty to discharge statutory obligations, can (often wrongly) militate against that approach being adopted. Similarly, the use of individual counselling can falter in the face of silence, or answers limited to 'OK' on the part of the adolescent being counselled. Confronted with these problems, forming groups of adolescents which can utilise the benefits of peer group influence, whilst maintaining a problem-centred approach, has to many social workers appeared to be the preferred solution. But in adopting this method there are two important factors which should be considered.

The first factor is that the role of the parents, and the relationships which they establish with their children, are crucially important. Many social workers having established a group of adolescents often seem to disregard contact with the family, rather than attempting to use groupwork as a basis for improving family relationships (Jones, 1979). However, groupwork with adolescents is no more the single 'right' response than any other, and it should be seen as one in a range of responses that might be required to help an adolescent, particularly where that response needs to involve 'significant others', such as the family. Some groupwork programmes and social work agencies have attempted to recognise this. Byng-Hall and Bruggen (1974) describe a family-based approach to work with adolescents in a psychiatric adolescent unit. They see the decision to admit to the unit as being crucial, and one which should not be removed from the family or person legally responsible for the adolescent. The work of the unit is concerned with attempting to recreate or affirm the family's authority over their own lives, rather than separate or destroy such responsibility, which is often one consequence of a reception into care.

The second major factor in working with an adolescent in a group is to appreciate something of his previous experience and at what level of personal development he operates. This is important for four reasons. First, it can help to locate groupwork programmes appropriately within the community. It might be important to create groups or facilitate contact with them at times which are appropriate to the adolescent. Perhaps the meeting place should be in premises or on territory which is familiar to the service receiver rather than to the service provider. Second, it is necessary to recognise different group needs at different stages of development. When is it best to create a mixed-sex group and when not? What differences in interests will there be between 12-year-olds and 16-year-olds? Third, we need to be aware that we should establish communication on a level which is understandable to the adolescent. This means using words and methods which are easily understood, and offering explanations for working in a group which can be perceived (and agreed upon) by all participants. Finally interests and activities can be used, where appropriate, which relate to the peer group culture of which the adolescent is a part. Therefore whether the groupwork programmes include a focus on keeping ferrets, playing football or watching speedway should be largely determined by the interests and enthusiasms of the adolescents. This does not mean that other areas of activity are excluded (indeed it might be an objective of the intervention to promote new interests), but that to pursue them successfully calls for additional support and encouragement. This might be gained by the charisma and personality with which a groupworker promotes those interests. On the other hand promoting interests needs to be done in such a way that the adolescent does not become an object of ridicule by his 'mates' for being involved in such unusual activities, and also the activities should be available and accessible to the adolescent after the groupwork programme has finished.

As stated earlier social groupwork is only one approach to problem solving, and the key as to whether or not it is adopted depends on the type of problem being tackled. Douglas (1976) and Heap (1979) both put forward reasons

for starting a group which can be combined into two simple
maxims: (1) it is the best means available at that particular
time for tackling a particular problem situation or issue,
and (2) by offering a groupwork response the participants
may actually be of help to each other. Before examining
these issues it is necessary to look at how groupwork with
adolescents has developed in Britain, because the kind of
groups being operated appear to be more a consequence of
historical accident rather than being planned on a basis of
identified need.

THE DEVELOPMENT OF GROUPWORK WITH ADOLESCENTS IN BRITAIN

The practice of groupwork with adolescents has had a long
if intermittent history. Octavia Hill in working with ragged
school children attempted to mobilise groups with the objective of creating and working in a co-operative toy factory
during the nineteenth century. The Quakers' model school
at Ackworth, established in 1779, relied heavily on peer
group leadership, with the older children teaching the
younger ones. Although varying groupwork models have
been used in psychiatric units, experimental schools, and
child-guidance clinics, it was not until the 1960s that a
broader development began to take place. Motivated by
news of projects in USA (see Advisory Council on the
Treatment of Offenders, 1962), with an increasing realisa-
tion of the inappropriateness of one-to-one casework with
adolescents who were inarticulate, and with the provision of
a small amount of funding (from the 1963 Children and Young
Persons Act), some new schemes began to operate. They
were later to find legislative support in the 1969 Children
and Young Persons Act under the banner of what has become
known as 'intermediate treatment'.
  One scheme at Pontefract in Yorkshire started in 1961
when a probation officer got together with the local Society
of Friends to find an alternative setting for work with a
group of about seven boys on Probation Orders. The club
was intended as a setting where those boys on the probation
officer's caseload could begin to develop 'meaningful relationships with adults and peers in an independent and secure
atmosphere where they can get satisfaction from socially
accepted challenges' (Rowntree, 1965). From this a large
project has now developed which employs five full-time

workers, and offers a range of community and groupwork
programmes, not only for adolescents but also for other
groups such as mums and toddlers (DHSS, 1977a).

The children's department also began to look at alternative methods of working. Packman, writing about Oxford-
shire Children's Department, observed that:

> Involvement with numbers of difficult teenagers also
> spurred the department into experiments with a wider
> range of treatment methods ... from 1960 onwards seve-
> ral mountain camps were arranged and teenagers in care
> were taught the rudiments of camping and climbing, under
> the leadership of a male child care officer and in the
> company of other members of staff. Even the Children's
> Officer visited the camps and was rememberd, 'in a bell
> tent, with more holes in it than a colander, trying to
> make sandwiches and keep them dry in a mountain thunder-
> storm'. The Curtis maxim of 'the personal element in
> child care as personified in the role of the Children's
> Officer' was apparently alive and well in the 1960s
> (Packman, 1975, pp. 108-9).

On a theoretical level various influences were apparent and,
despite the work of authorities such as Docker Drysdale
(1968) in Britain, many of these came from the USA. Here
groupwork possessed a history which stretched back to the
1920s when the Western Reserve University began to offer
a groupwork course based on the work of the community
settlements. In the post-war period the impact of groupwork on different client categories was examined, and for
adolescents this was represented by the publication of
Coyle's 'Groupwork with American Youth' in 1948.

By the 1960s groupwork had become sufficiently established to be included on a variety of social work training
courses in Britain but its practical potential was still
largely seen as being limited to psychiatric settings. However some authors (and particularly Konopka, 1963) began
to propose a much more dynamic form of intervention, which
moved away from the static 'T' Group style and the psychotherapeutic orientation of Foulkes and Anthony (1962), and
therefore had more applicability to social work with children and adolescents.

Since the 1960s one of the primary influences on development of social groupwork with adolescents has been the
(limited) growth of intermediate treatment. Indeed the two
areas have become so intertwined that the terms 'groupwork
with adolescents' and 'intermediate treatment' are often used

as if inter-changeable by the professional and laymen alike.
However they are not the same, the former being a description of a method of social work with a particular client
group, and the latter a generic term for a range of methods,
resources and programmes. This confusion of intermediate
treatment and groupwork has arisen for a variety of reasons. Although intermediate treatment has been conceptua-
lised as a range of provision from community-based youth
clubs to residential care, in practice the majority of work
has centred on the once-a-week activity-based group.
Baldwin outlines the 'small group model' of intermediate
treatment in detail:

1 Membership of 8 to 12 adolescents, within a two to
   three year age band between 10 and 17. Mixed or
   single sex.
2 Two to four adult workers, sufficient to provide a variety of adult models and close individual relationships.
3 Group members referred by social workers, probation
   officers, E.W.O.'s and school staff. Majority under
   supervision or care orders, but some regarded as at
   risk, either of delinquent behaviour or care proceed-
   ings.
4 Group meets once or twice weekly for two or three
   hours but also has some shared residential experience
   in periods of two to five days. Overall length of group
   either set at the start, between six and twelve months,
   or open ended.
5 Members of the group will be involved with adults in
   planning the programme, and in the general management
   of the group.
6 The programme will include a range of activities, some
   centre-based, others using community resources. It
   may include some form of community service, self-help
   project and/or the use of creative activities, such as
   art, drama or music. The programme will normally
   involve discussion, either at set times or spontaneous-
   ly, and this will focus on the shared experiences of the
   group and of individual problems and development
(Baldwin, 1977, p. 7).

Whilst such a model is so open-ended as to encompass
more than one style of groupwork intervention, it still
offers an indication of how groupwork within intermediate
treatment has tended to develop. A further reason for confusion between groupwork with adolescents and intermediate
treatment is due to the growth and domination of the statu-

tory agencies, particularly social services, within social
work, and any developments by these agencies has often
overshadowed developments in other fields. Groupwork
with adolescents has taken place elsewhere, such as in
ROSLA projects (White and Brockington, 1978), therapeutic
communities (Wills, 1971), and voluntary counselling
schemes (Truckle and Schardt, 1975), but because of the
isolation of these projects lessons derived from them can
easily be overlooked by the mainstream agencies.

The problem is that whilst groupwork has been stimulated
by the growth of intermediate treatment, this has also had
the effect of narrowing the definition and potentiality of
what that work could be. In addition, because this area
has been a new and difficult one for social workers to
master, some of the adolescent groups formed have often
had a closer resemblance to 'playgroups' rather than 'work
groups'.

Nevertheless by adopting a groupwork approach social
work and social workers have taken a hesitant step towards
utilising the strengths of both the peer group and the community in helping adolescents in trouble. As Macklennan
and Felsenfeldt argue, such a step can present valuable
opportunities:

Small groups provide a miniature real life situation
which can be utilised for the study and change of behaviour. In groups people expose their typical patterns of
operation. New ways of dealing with situations can be
learned in action. New skills in human relations can be
developed, current problems resolved, and standards and
values re-examined and altered. The group skilfully
conducted can provide a mirror in which the group member
can evolve a new concept of himself, test this out in
action with his fellows, and find new models for identification (Macklennan and Felsenfeldt, 1968, p. 51).

PREPARING AND FORMING GROUPS

Earlier in this chapter, two reasons for adopting a group
approach were offered: first, the group was the best means
available at that time for coping with an issue or a problem,
and second, that within the group its members could actually help each other. Frequently these simple maxims are
ignored and either groups are formed for inappropriate
reasons or else they are asked to achieve impossible tasks.

In the case of the former it is not uncommon to hear of projects being initiated to increase the experience and status of social work agencies or to offer students an opportunity 'to take part in a group'. In the instance of groups being asked to achieve too much, then the reason is normally that a group is viewed in isolation as the only response to a problem rather than being integrated with other services and provision. For an adolescent who has been rejected by his school, faces relationship problems with his family, lives in poor housing and in a highly delinquent neighbourhood, then a groupwork programme is only one of several services that should be provided.

The DHSS booklet 'Intermediate Treatment: Planning for Action' lists a variety of aims and objectives for adolescent groups:

Aims

1 Provide opportunities to (a) learn to interact with a greater variety of people; (b) perform and experience different roles in the group: leading, following, cooperative behaviour, competitive behaviour etc.

2 These aspects are important for individuals who have been isolated from normal opportunities because of deviance, lack of confidence, illness, handicaps etc.

3 Groups can be helpful for people to test out their impact on others.

4 Group control is often more realistic, acceptable, and more effective than individual control, especially in adolescent groups.

5 The group situation can dilute the dependence of a one-to-one relationship and break the trend of the 'helper-helped' situation of casework.

Potential outcomes of group experiences

1 Relief through expression of feelings.

2 Desired behavioural change.

3 Improvement in social relationships.

4 Group cohesiveness and a sense of belonging.

5 Self understanding and understanding of others.

6 Obtaining information.

7 Social and/or emotional contact (DHSS, 1977b, p. 25).

Whilst such a list should not be seen as exclusive it can be an aid to the worker in trying to define objectives. The necessity of this kind of preparation and thought before running any group is emphasised by Douglas:

To take into consideration as many factors as possible before the group is actually convened means clearing ideas to the point that a groupworker has got a reasonable certainty about what he intends to do. This can only be beneficial especially when contracts are made for the simple reason that the groupworker may be faced with the task of 'selling' what he has to offer to a relatively dis- believing client. If his own ideas and values are hazy, then he will not be convincing (Douglas, 1976, p. 41).

To assist in preparing a groupwork programme several authors have offered a 'checklist' approach (Douglas, 1976; Hodge, 1977; Jones and Kerslake, 1979). Most of these lists involve the worker in questioning what exactly it is that he or she intends to do, on a basis that detailed plan- ning increases both the groupworker(s) and the members security. A common feature of the 'checklists' is that they highlight four key areas of preparation:

1 deciding the purpose of the group;
2 selecting group members;
3 deciding upon the frequency and type of contact;
4 examining the relationship of the group to the social work agency and to the community.

Deciding, defining and agreeing upon a clear objective or purpose of what you are attempting is of particular impor- tance when establishing a 'formed' adolescent group. Without clarity about objectives it becomes difficult to re- solve the other issues mentioned above, such as selecting the members of the group if you do not know why you are selecting them. But having established a central purpose (which needs to be understood by members and leaders alike) does not mean that alternative secondary goals should be ignored, or that they should not be allowed to develop as the group begins to function. Hodge argues that the worker in all instances should avoid establishing covert objectives:

The groupworker should not normally be drawn into de- fining aims which are to be concealed from the members, e.g. a group for adoptive parents convened to discuss child care principles should not be used to assess the suitability of the members as adoptive parents unless such an intention has been explicitly stated to the group members (Hodge, 1977, p. 9).

The second key area, concerning the purposeful selec- tion of members, is sometimes avoided for both positive and negative reasons. Positively this occurs when the worker becomes involved with a 'natural' peer group, or works with a group who have been involved in offending together, or when the group self-selects by coming to the social work

office together   for an individual interview (as described by
Heap, 1977).   Negatively, however, selection is mishand-
led when a worker is only allowed to lead a group if a pre-
ponderance of clients from his caseload are included, or
when a random collection of all adolescent clients are put
together because 'it seems to be the easiest way of dealing
with them'.   Where a group is to be purposefully selected
then various criteria need to be considered.   What age
range is appropriate?   What kind of sex balance should be
achieved?   How many members?   Who actually does the
selecting?   These are all important questions.   With adolescents it is often maturational age that is much more important than chronological age, and in selecting for an adolescent group one should also take into account Dunphy's peer
group development categorisation that was discussed
earlier.

   In the third key area of the checklists, issues such as
when, where and how frequently the group meets have a
practical relevance and also an emotional importance concerned with providing security.   This is especially important when it is considered that many of the adolescents in
contact with social workers are made to face uncertainty
every day.   Just being clear about where and when the
group will take place can be a vital first step in building
relationships and establishing trust.

   The final key area of importance in preparing to operate
a group concerns its relationship to the agency and to the
community of which it is a part.   Willson writes that:

   The negotiation of an adequate contract within the agency
   is a necessary prerequisite for the staff of a groupwork
   project that is to be run within that agency: only then can
   the subsequent negotiations with co-workers and clients
   have any application.   The experience of that negotiation,
   whether it results in a modified groupwork project or
   none, will be invaluable and illuminating to all involved
   (Willson, 1978, p. 13).

Having established a clear contract with the agency over
what resources will be needed, and the relationship of the
group to the remainder of the agency's work with adolescents (e.g. in the case of a supervision order, who holds
the statutory responsibility when groupworker and case-
worker are not the same person), there are still other
agency-related factors to consider.   These include the
method of recording or monitoring to be used, the form of
supervision or consultation which will be available for the

groupworkers and how much information your colleagues
need to make referrals and to understand what you are
doing.

The role of the group in the community is a much more
intangible idea to take into account. Two considerations
might be: what happens to group members after each session and at the end of the groupwork programme? If the
group is an intensive and emotionally demanding experience
for the adolescent, but nevertheless still based within the
community, then how much support will the adolescent need
at the end of each session, or indeed how will the session
end, so that each individual can leave as a 'whole' person?
This is particularly true where confrontational techniques
are being used. The worker will need to take into account
the nature and kind of confrontation that the adolescent
might also be experiencing at home. Other issues involving the community are: what do those outside the group see
it as achieving, what happens to the members at the end of
the groupwork programme, and what are the attitudes of
other adults, such as teachers, to the adolescent and to the
group? The ability of the adolescent to understand what
he is involved in, and for other interested parties to perceive the group as being beneficial, can be essential in
determining its ultimate success.

LEADERSHIP IN ADOLESCENT GROUPS

One issue not yet mentioned is the leadership role of the
social worker(s) and this requires special consideration as
it is a continuing feature throughout the life of the group.

In considering leadership style, potential group leaders
need to ask two questions: what is the relationship of the
leader to the group and how does one see oneself as a
leader? In thinking about the relationship of the leader to
the group questions arise concerning how many leaders are
needed, are they involved in selecting the group members,
what kind of leadership is appropriate, and how well, if
co-workers are involved, can the leaders work together?
But leadership also involves an assessment by the groupworker of his or her own ability. By asking what makes
you uncomfortable, how directive do you like to be, and
how do you respond to tension in a group, can help to
improve one's leadership skills. Developing a comfortable
and appropriate leadership response for many social work-

ers can be both a difficult, and sometimes frightening task,
as the quote below illustrates:

Here is an example of a student social worker in a training situation with a group of boys 'at risk' aged 12:
'As soon as the building was opened to the boys Andy
bounded in as if possessed. He swung an ancient hockey
stick at the walls, doors and light switches as he went.
Once brought to a halt by the end of the building two
naked light bulbs were too much of a temptation. He
smashed them. The student was very angry and began
to manhandle him towards the entrance saying, "You don't
come here to do that, I'm putting you out for this".'
Several weeks later:
'Andy was working at the bench. In too much of a hurry
he split the wood he was nailing. Swearing violently,
he struck at the wood, then turning to a naked light
smashed the bulb, showering the other boys present with
splinters. The worker who was in the room laughed and
said "Accidents will happen".'
From a treatment standpoint both reactions were wrong,
although entirely understandable in a training situation.
In the first example the student should have allowed for
the pent-up frustration Andy brought with him. He
should have used first his relationship with Andy in a
much less emotional manner and later consulted the group
of boys as a whole in negotiating standards of acceptable
behaviour. In the second example, he should have reminded Andy of the limits on behaviour previously nego-
tiated. It can be argued that on the first occasion the
student was confirming Andy's already established hostility towards adults and on the second he was underlin-
ing the acceptability of anti-social behaviour (Alpin and
Bamber, 1973, p. 7).

The incident described above shows that developing
appropriate worker responses in groups is not always an
easy task. The worker who is neither in control of the
group, nor, more importantly, in control of himself, can
easily fall into an inconsistent leadership style. Heron
(1975) talks of 'degenerative' forms of leadership style and
in groupwork with adolescents there are various ways in
which these can emerge. Group members running 'amok'
or a completely 'laissez-faire' leadership becomes inaccu-
rately interpreted as 'democratic'. Dogmatic or authoritarian leadership, which often leaves the group members
with no participation in decision making, becomes expressed
by the degenerative leader as 'controlling' or 'structured'.

Willson describes the skills and limitations of a team of groupworkers as being the product of:
1 The personality of the worker(s),
2 The nature of the co-worker relationship in the case of there being more than one staff member, and
3 The agency from which the staff team work (Willson, 1978, p. 12).
Despite concentrating on several of the points mentioned above, much of the impact that the worker can make centres on the personality, involvement and commitment of that individual. Whilst such factors cannot be taught, where they already exist good support and supervision can undoubtedly help to maximise them.

Being clear about the purpose and aims of the group, and having established a comfortable relationship with your co-worker(s) can all help in enabling concentration to be devoted towards the group's members. Even where this has been achieved contentious issues can still arise, and one of the most common is that of control. The British Association of Social Workers, in discussing the development of groupwork with adolescents, sees control as: 'largely exercised in a group by the group workers themselves. It is they who define what is acceptable and non-acceptable forms of behaviour. Where youngsters exceed limits set, difficulties should be dealt with firmly and on the spot' (BASW, 1977, p. 21).

Although on occasions such firmness may be necessary to control potentially damaging or dangerous situations for group members, or else to reaffirm the direction of the group, as an overall leadership strategy the statement creates several difficulties. First, by the groupworkers appearing authoritarian, or by making the rules, it not only denies any potential the adolescent may have to do this, but also confirms a world view of adults as 'holding all the cards'. It is also unlikely to produce a situation which generates trust or relationship building. Second, as Thorpe points out:
Rule breaking is normal in adolescence and it is even necessary if experimentation with roles and relationships is to occur. In this sense all adolescents are emotionally disturbed.... Inevitably therefore limits will be exceeded and it is the manner in which rule breaking is handled, that constitutes much of the therapy in the intermediate treatment setting (Thorpe, 1977, p. 19).
Confronted by this problem, workers often attempt to

develop a democratic ethos of rule- and decision-making within the group, although in practice this often results in semi-anarchy or in the workers still making the decisions, but denying that they do so. Democratic decision-making only takes place when the knowledge and information necessary is available to all; in this context 'democracy needs to be learnt' (White and Brockington, 1978). One group illustrated this by the leaders asking the group members to jointly plan the menu for a proposed camping trip. The initial responses that came back were clearly impracticable, not because the adolescents were trying to be 'difficult' but because they did not possess essential information. They did not appreciate what could be cooked on a camping stove, how long this took, or have the ability to weigh up the benefits of a quick meal leaving time for other activities. The workers then planned the first trip, but over succeeding weeks they gradually devolved the responsibility back to the members. By the time the final session was reached not only did the group members plan the menus and cook the food, but they were also able to make suggestions as to how the food could be prepared in a better way than the workers had previously considered.

The most effective means of control within adolescent groups relies on establishing group norms of behaviour which are acceptable to all, and using controls which are already in existence. Norms are partly established by those values and behaviour patterns that all the group members bring with them, and partly enforced by the mutually agreed goals that the group is attempting to achieve. Rather than the worker laying down the rules, discussing with the adolescents what boundaries the group needs is much more likely to be successful. Northern writes that:

Since norms are usually based on agreement among members, the need for personal power to enforce the norms is reduced and responsibility for enforcement is shared among the members. Norms that are accepted and complied with, become intrinsically rewarding, thus reducing the need for external control. Norms thus provide a means for controlling behaviour without entailing the cost and uncertainties involved in the unrestrained use of interpersonal power (Northern, 1969, p. 35).

In developing the controls that the adolescents already possess the social worker may well find them to be more powerful and beneficial than previously thought. It should always be considered before using personal intervention

whether the group can regulate disruptive behaviour itself
and if not, why not? For instance, Peter Marsh offers an
example of two football fans regulating the propensity of
another to boast about 'terrace' violence:

Fan A: When we played Everton in the F.A. Cup I spent
two weeks in hospital, I got seven busted ribs
and a broken nose.

Fan B: No, that's exaggerating. The young fellas, you
know they're giving each other verbal and that,
you know, and they're running each other down;
that's all harmless fun you know, even if they
sort of have a little chase and chase one another
round the grounds.... But when it comes to
people bringing out knives, that's out of order.

Fan A: But it's changed; it's changed, everything comes
out now. Alright, fair enough, when we go
away, I'll admit it, I do people in the eyes with
ammonia, so what? Right? I got done at Everton, and since I've been there I've carried that
ammonia with me all the time. There's no way I
go away without that ammonia.

Fan C: Where is it now then?

Fan A: Today I haven't got it, right?

Fan C: Aah, I don't believe you, I don't believe you.
If you take it everywhere why ain't you got it
today?

Fan A: 'Cos I haven't been home to get it. Straight,
that's the truth (Marsh, 1978, pp. 74-5).

THE CONTENT OF GROUPWORK PROGRAMMES

Having decided upon an objective or reason for using a
group approach with adolescents means that part of the task
of formulating an appropriate programme is complete. The
objectives set for, or by, the group should guide and influence the process and method by which they are to be
achieved. For example, if the task of the group relates to
education and has the objectives of (a) improving school
attendance, (b) helping to make education more relevant to
those receiving it, and (c) providing opportunities to 'catch
up' on previous school work, then the content of the programme should be determined by these objectives. Part of
the work will have features common to many groups, such
as encouraging members to help and support each other, but

having enabled individuals to work together and to draw benefits from being a group the focus returns to the educational goals. The techniques to be used might include individual reading tuition (by using everyday items such as newspapers and bus timetables as source learning material), offering work experience and day visits to factories, role-playing teacher/pupil incidents, and focusing on option bargaining over attendance.

Despite the logic behind such an approach, many groups fail to link objectives and programme content. This sometimes results in a crazy situation where beneficial methods are being used, but towards an unachievable objective, or alternatively appropriate objectives are set but these are unrelated to the method used in the group. Another dilemma is where the group centres on one limited objective and, rather than being a place where experiment can occur between adult and adolescent over commonly held goals, the group remains fixed on one task, such as organising a camping trip or a particular kind of activity. This is not to decry the value of 'activity', but activity-based tasks need to be seen as a means to the end set for the group rather than as an end in their own right.

Vinter (1967) describes the use of activities in groups and the potential effect that they might have. He also lays emphasis on developing sequences of activities which have meaning in terms of the objectives of the group. However, in the sometimes apparent flight (through intermediate treatment) of field social workers away from casework with adolescents, the need to communicate with the adolescent about personal problems or worries often seems to have been ignored. Whilst it is possible to sympathise with what has become an almost audible sigh of relief from both workers and adolescents alike at having been 'let out of the office', the adults are still social workers and their adolescent clients are still often facing problems which need resolution. In an intensive group, where there is a high degree of worker/group member contact, discussion of problems need not always be formalised, but in less intensive settings important personal concerns and issues can easily be lost in the rush from mountain climbing to pony trekking. In these situations group workers often fall back on providing a set discussion time, despite the members frequently perceiving such sessions as 'boring'. Waterhouse, in commenting on a groupwork project for adolescents who had been involved in delinquency, comments:

discussion proved the most difficult (out of the methods of role play, activities and discussion) to sustain. It was not easy to get young people, many of whom had quite well-developed talents for acting-out and disruption, to sit and discuss a topic like 'what I think about school' or 'how I get on with my parents' (Waterhouse, 1978, p. 132).

What is often ignored is that discussion can be promoted outside set discussion times. Role play and group exercises are equally as valid a means of promoting discussion as 'straight talk'. In addition they also encourage greater group participation. The task of the group worker is to make space, and to act as an enabler and as a non-condemnatory listener when there is a need for discussion to occur. This is an important but far from easy task to perform, as Waterhouse again illustrates:

Role play and games proved to be ways of ensuring a much higher degree of participation and involvement, although these too were open to the possibility of disruption by more wayward group members.... Observing these activities, it became clear that the major task for the group worker was to use the material which was brought up. Was the activity an end in itself or was it a means to an end? For example one group re-enacted a robbery which involved an assault on a night watchman. This was performed with great gusto and involvement, but little time was then given over to a discussion of the issues and attitudes involved.... The issue is in a sense a technical one, well known to teachers working with the medium of role play and simulation; that of how to make the transition from the simulated experience to a discussion of the feelings and issues which the simulation has raised (Waterhouse, 1978, p. 132).

In designing the content of groupwork programmes workers need to be concerned with not only developing planned activities or tasks, but also to be aware of the potential presented by unplanned incidents. Unplanned events need not always have an unplanned response! It is possible to anticipate some issues which may face the group, such as bullying, members not arriving at a scheduled meeting place, or transport arrangements breaking down. The task for the workers is to discuss before such events occur their potential responses, and possibly even to role play possible reactions.

During the life of any adolescent group learning poten-

tial is also available in the 'daily events' or routine activities of the group, such as preparing a meal.   White and
Brockington (1978) describe a trip with one group member
to a department store to buy nails which developed into a
social skills and reading exercise lasting 20 minutes.   If
a window is broken in premises used by the group then it
is not just a situation demanding the exertion of some authority by the group leader as it can also promote group discussion ('who pays?'; 'who is to mend it?'), group cohesion ('we will all mend it together'), social skills ('where
and how do you buy glass, putty, nails?'), and craft skills
('how do you use putty?'; 'how many nails should be knocked
in?'; 'what kind of glass do we need?').   Casual remarks
and comments can also be focused upon when they offer the
potential for group discussion and analysis of problems.
Norman, in discussing a project at 870 House in Birmingham, describes the technique of 'freezing' important
moments in a group's life:

> The purpose is to examine in detail exactly what is hap-
> pening, to try to identify what is going wrong (or right)
> and to try to spot what has 'triggered' off the situation.
> The 'trigger', when identified, may well give the clue as
> to the most appropriate method of intervening or tackling
> the problem.
>
> When you decide to freeze and analyse – stop whatever
> is happening (e.g. get the group sitting down together,
> stop the role play session, stop the counselling session),
> then suggest to the participant(s) that together they ex-
> amine that particular session in depth.   Then, if they
> are willing to co-operate, get them to really examine the
> situation as thoroughly as possible.   Keep on repeating
> the pattern to the member(s) as it becomes clear so that
> they see the situation more clearly.   Then try, together,
> to identify the 'trigger'.   Remember that for this process
> to work effectively, everyone participating must them-
> selves see and understand what has happened and what
> has 'triggered off' the situation.
>
> Freezing and analysing usually occurs in one of three
> situations at 870:
> (a) The individual situation, where a member of staff and
>   one 'client' freeze and analyse together.
> (b) The group situation, where several people work toge-
>   ther to analyse a situation.
> (c) The Hot Seat, where one member invites the group to
>   discuss him/her in depth with his/her active partici-
>   pation (Norman, 1977, pp. 12-13).

The opportunities for learning and development in a group presented by ordinary events and conversations are often best handled by a worker when using a less than overt leadership style. Leading by example and attempting to be the 'best group member' rather than the direct leader are two ways in which this can be accomplished. Using processes generated by the group also offers learning potential. Button (1974) describes how techniques such as physical contact, action research, and psycho-drama can encourage mutual support and sharing in a group, and he states that:

> It is very impressive to see how rapidly young people will share the group worker's role. Individual youngsters may sometimes lead a phase of questioning of one of their colleagues, and as they learn to recognise the need for help and to offer help, this soon begins to flow beyond the confines of the group.... When a group of youngsters reach this stage, support for one another through discussion and action may continue outside the group meetings (Button, 1974, p. 78).

Using the processes of the group facilitates the achievement of its goals and is therefore not only a desirable objective, but can also be a rewarding way of working. It is often all too easy in a group for the leader to take over and to complete the task rather than to encourage the involvement of the group members or to speak, rather than to create opportunities for others in the group to express their ideas and opinions.

OTHER SETTINGS FOR GROUPWORK WITH
ADOLESCENTS

So far this chapter has concentrated on the role of the field social worker in establishing and working with formed groups of adolescent 'clients'. In addition it has attempted to place that role in both an historical and peer group context. However, there are several other settings in social care agencies which have the potential to use, or are engaged in, groupwork with adolescents. The most obvious of these are residential establishments, schools and youth clubs. There has also been the influence of groupwork in settings such as pyschiatric adolescent units. With the development of intermediate treatment some groupwork projects have begun to explore the overlap between these agencies and field social work.

Although in the residential establishments, schools and
youth clubs the context of work is often the group, this does
not necessarily mean that what is happening is groupwork.
The difference might appear semantic, but groupwork calls
for an attempt to consciously use the processes within the
group. Therefore whilst residential homes or schools
might argue that all the work they do is groupwork, there
are many instances when it could be more useful to define
and develop further small groupwork within the larger setting. The limited extent to which this has been accomplished was illustrated by a government report on hostels
for young people (DHSS, 1975) which found that only four
of the forty residential hostels studied showed any evidence
of using groupwork.

In his study of secondary schools Hargreaves (1967)
asserted that teachers frequently underestimated or ignored
the power and influence of the peer group in the school, but
several education experiments have attempted to respond to
and develop the small adolescent groups as a means of improving the quality of education. Whilst the school has
considerable potential in terms of the amount of contact it
has with adolescents, encouraging the use of groupwork as
a means of learning is not always easy. Perceiving personal growth and development as learning is difficult when
teachers more readily associate learning with facts and
information giving. Over the last ten years some of these
problems have diminished with the increased attention devoted to curriculum development. There has been some
movement towards using group exercises in the classroom,
team teaching, and developing the 'form' group into something more than just a random group of adolescents collected together by virtue either of their chronological age or
their surname. Clark (1968), for instance, discusses the
use of simulation games and role-play in the classroom.
But despite this, approaches that take the group beyond the
periphery of academic education and into the realm of social
education have mainly occurred in experimental and 'alternative education' projects. Grunsell (1976) describes one
scheme in a small education unit:

> In small structural groups of never more than seven, we
> try to fit our work to the children's needs at the time.
> Because the centre is small, we can have a flexible time-
> table and change it week by week. According to the
> children's interests and concerns - whether it be job ·
> opportunities, social security, history or biology - we

can adapt our curriculum to cope with it, something a large comprehensive cannot do. In all our teaching, we try to reach back into the children's homes. If a particular child expresses problems with regard to his parents, say, then that too can be drawn into the teaching situation if he wants it to be (Grunsell, 1976, p. 11).

The residential setting partially mirrors that of the community by presenting two areas of working, the 'natural' group (the group of all residents and staff in day to day interaction) and the 'formed' group (where specific individuals may be brought together to achieve a particular task or objective). Payne outlines six areas where a knowledge of group behaviour and a need to use group skills are appropriate in the 'natural' residential group:

1 In developing and managing the 'natural resources' of group living.
2 In identifying, managing and mitigating the many tensions and stresses encountered in daily living.
3 In facilitating the integration of the newcomer to the residential setting, and correspondingly, in helping him to prepare for departure from the setting.
4 In providing opportunities for personal development and life enrichment.
5 In helping residents find solutions to the interpersonal and other life problems that have often been the cause of their admission into care.
6 In helping residential staff to exercise constructive and creative leadership, in particular through a continuous process of appraisal and review of the happenings of residential life (Payne, 1978, p. 60).

In constructing 'formed' groups in a residential setting considerations additional to those raised earlier in this chapter should be taken into account. There is increased concern over confidentiality and what will happen to information gained during group sessions. Pairings formed in the group are more likely to be influenced by what happens outside and thereby subject to pressure. It might also be harder for group leaders to cope with the duality of their role of balancing authority with care. Tutt examines several of these issues, but concludes that the group he observed in a community home possessed the advantages that:

it made the staff more aware of the boys' problems, and therefore more likely and more able to help the boys individually to deal with their problems. The groups were also important in intensifying existing personal relation-

ships between staff and boys by showing the boys another
side of an authority figure (Tutt, 1974, p. 79).

The Youth and Community Service also offers many
opportunities for small groupwork with adolescents. A
long history of encouraging leadership from within the
peer group, and the provision of varying kinds of residential courses, illustrate these opportunities. Yet there are
still many areas of youth work which are based on activity-
orientated youth centres where the skills of the worker are
more often directed into providing coffee, teaching karate
and maintaining the premises, rather than on personal relationships. Eggleston suggests that:

The concept of the Youth Service as being able to provide
most things, for most young people, is possibly something
of an anachronism. It may be that we no longer need to
try to serve the needs of, say, many of the young people
who are successful and well catered for in schools
(Eggleston, 1975, p. 202).

For the worker in the youth club the dilemma might be in
dividing time between the needs of a small group and the
larger membership, or alternatively between neighbourhood-
and centre-based work, but where the adolescent has rejected more 'authoritarian' adults such as the teacher or the
social worker, a considerable responsibility rests on the
youth worker. The youth worker may be the only person
able to deal with the problems that are being presented, and
offering traditional activities and minimal worker/member
contact would not be appropriate. As Button argues:

If young people are to be given real opportunities for
personal development, they will need to be caught up in
the kind of experience that is likely to extend them. The
time that many of them spend in their clubs can be desultory, repetitive in content, boring and stilting rather
than extending. Altogether, it may represent a suspen-
sion of movement rather than a time of personal development. We are not likely to be able to offer young people
the opportunities they require unless we can considerably
intensify their experience beyond what can be provided by
the large and looser organisation. In order to introduce
this element of greater intensity we shall need to work
through small groups within the larger institution
(Button, 1974, p. 141).

Therefore in residential establishments, schools and
the youth service there is much potential for developing
groupwork, but to do so successfully calls for relaxing the

boundaries and divisions between the services provided by
the differing agencies and in the varying settings.   The
problems concerning inter-professional communication have
been discussed in Chapter four, but in terms of advancing
groupwork as a method of work with adolescents it would
seem that benefits can be gained by offering a service which
is more responsive to the adolescents' needs by bringing
together workers from different disciplines.

CONCLUSION

The practice of working with groups of adolescents is, as
has been illustrated, subject to many influences.   For the
social worker there are choices about whether to increase
involvement with the 'natural' peer group or to work in a
'formed' group, what kind of setting and intensity of contact
should be offered, and whether it might not be more appropriate to encourage teachers or youth workers to extend the
boundaries of their work.   Underlying these decisions are
the constraints imposed by that worker's agency, the community, and even the adolescent and their family.   Despite
the obvious growth, both in the amount and range of groupwork with adolescents over the last ten years, there are
still many social work agencies that regard it as the social
workers' personal part-time hobby and somehow irrelevant
to the 'proper work'.   However agencies also have a responsibility to encourage professional practice, and in this
respect many have been lax in offering consultation and support to social workers practising groupwork.   The intention in this chapter has not been to promote working in small
groups over and above any other method, but to illustrate
where, how, and why groups can and have been developed.
The response of the social worker should always be in discovering and understanding the needs being presented before
deciding on method of work.

Chapter seven

Neighbourhood work
with adolescents

Ray Jones

/This paper continues the theme already established in
this book of looking at 'normal' adolescent development, and
then exploring possible problems for adolescents and social
work responses to these problems. The focus for this
chapter is the adolescent within his neighbourhood. The
paper examines the importance of the neighbourhood to the
adolescent, and the meaning which 'neighbourhood' has for
him. It then discusses how some neighbourhoods may predispose adolescents towards trouble, and hence ultimately
towards becoming social work clients. The final sections
of the paper describe how the concept of 'neighbourhood'
may have relevance to the philosophy of social work, and
how social workers might use a neighbourhood perspective
to enhance their practice./

THE NEIGHBOURHOOD AND ADOLESCENTS

Neighbourhood work is a fairly recent innovation within
many contemporary social work agencies. It still has the
status of being 'experimental', and developments in this
aspect of social work practice remain infrequent and insecure. Cut-backs in funding, in staffing levels, or increasing (statutory) responsibilities in other areas of work,
often result in neighbourhood projects being axed. It is
not therefore surprising that much of the innovatory work
in this area has been accomplished by voluntary agencies.
This has been especially true for neighbourhood work with
adolescents. It has been voluntary agencies like the
Youth Development Trust in Manchester and the Young Volunteer Force Foundation (now the Community Projects

165

Foundation) which have been in the forefront of adopting a neighbourhood-based approach to working with young people. But what has neighbourhood work to offer adolescents? Is it relevant for them?

Chapter two suggested that adolescence is a time when young people are working at establishing their own adult identity. This requires a movement away from a dependence on their parents. One characteristic of this movement is a change in their behaviour. They spend less time at home with parents and, instead, their leisure time is mainly focused on activity outside the home in the company of their peers (Willmott, 1966; Rose and Marshall, 1974). Peers provide the support, status, and a tenuous security which was previously provided by parents. Peers partially replace parents as the adolescent's membership and reference groups.

Acceptance into the membership group of peers, and the award of a desired peer group status, is based on attitude and behaviour. The required attitudes and behaviours to achieve high status in the peer group vary from culture to culture, from social class to social class, and from time to time. Hargreaves (1967) has illustrated how in the 'A' streams of a secondary school, hard work, academic achievement, and conformity to teachers' values were rewarded by the classroom peer group. In the lower streams, however, these same attitudes and behaviour were shunned and those exhibiting them were ostracised or bullied. This difference between academic streams increased during the secondary school years. This is of some importance as school is one of the major life experiences for younger adolescents, and the school may be one of the major neighbourhood resources available to them. In this context it has been argued that some schools may encourage, or at least not discourage, delinquency and truanting, whilst at the same time producing few academically successful pupils (Power, 1967; Reynolds, 1976).

Hargreaves also noted that, especially for those in the lower academic streams, peer group status was largely determined by one's performance in leisure-time activities. It has been argued that particularly within working-class cultures there is an orientation towards activity which is exciting and immediately rewarding (Miller, 1958). Many adolescents are influenced by this ethos and leisure time for them is about seeking fun, excitement and immediate acceptance amongst their peers (Jones and Walter, 1978). This leisure time is often unstructured and unplanned, reflecting the lack of organisation and aspiration in the life of many adolescents. Their aspirations have already been stunted by the real prospects of limited income, limited job satis-faction and abundant insecurity in adult life (Willis, 1977). Matza (1964) has described how in 'drifting around' adoles-cents can become involved in delinquency and many studies of detached youth work illustrate the unstructured, apparent-ly aimless nature of leisure for many adolescents (Morse, 1965; Goetschius and Tash, 1967; Marchant and Smith, 1977).

The neighbourhood, therefore, is of importance to the adolescent, and has meaning for him, in four ways. The neighbourhood provides a venue for outside-home peer group activity where the adolescent can be away from parental scrutiny and supervision. It provides a readily accessible playground and leisure base. As such it provides a forum for the peer group, a place where one knows one can meet friends as an informal arrangement requiring no pre-plan-ning or organisation. This reflects the free-floating friendship groups who have no long-term commitment to any particular friends or activity. To some extent one's con-ception of one's neighbourhood provides the link between these dynamic, changing leisure groups and activities. One's subjective perceptions of territory and space, what you have learned to be safe ground or your own patch, sets parameters on the settings in which you meet with friends. But this is more a reflection of the life of the younger adol-escent for, as one community worker told me, the older adolescent may 'live in the neighbourhood but not be a part of it'. They go out of the neighbourhood to work, to places of entertainment, and to see their girlfriends or boyfriends. They often have their own means of transport, a motorbike or an old car. They may only come home to sleep. This image of the older adolescent becoming detached from his neighbourhood is echoed by Baldock: 'Adolescents who are beginning to establish their independence from their families are likely to be least attached to their neighbourhoods and to be attracted by peer-group activities that may take place some distance away from home' (Baldock, 1974, p. 44).

However, for the younger adolescents the territory which is yours may be a source of deprivation or opportunities. Parker (1974) described how in Liverpool tenement blocks adolescents make fun and excitement through involvement in delinquency, especially at the time of his study through joy

riding and stealing car radios. This is an environment
which has to be made exciting and stimulating. Gill's
(1977) account of life in 'Luke Street' further highlights
this picture of a drab environment being made exciting by
events which the kids create for themselves ... events
which can escalate into delinquency or be amplified by the
reactions and perceptions of others, such as neighbours
and the police, into 'disturbance' and 'trouble' (Gill, 1976).
One 13-year-old boy recently said to me that he disliked the
police because 'if you're having a bit of fun they always
stop you' (see also Corrigan, 1979). Fun for him had been
throwing stones through the windows of a disused railway
station. He now anticipates another court appearance after
being arrested by the Transport Police. However there
is another side to this picture. The police, for instance,
can also be seen as protectors by those adolescents who
are socially isolated or are not members of the more challenging local peer groups. Another lad, living in the same
neighbourhood as the boy above, said that policemen care
about you so that 'if people are getting you, like a gang of
kids with knives, they stop it'. Hence the neighbourhood
can also sometimes appear hostile to the adolescent and
does not necessarily always seem friendly.

THE NEIGHBOURHOOD AND TROUBLE

The quotations above from two adolescents show that a
neighbourhood can be experienced differently by different
people. There is also a suggestion that some neighbourhoods may predispose some adolescents towards trouble,
especially trouble as defined as law breaking. It is possible to discuss neighbourhoods which seem to encourage or
foster trouble in terms of their physical design and geographical location. One also needs to look at the reputation the neighbourhood may have, both for those who live
outside and those inside it, and to look at the localised
subculture which may lead to or result from this reputation.
    One form of trouble which is popularly associated with
adolescents is vandalism. The stereotype of the vandal is
the adolescent male throwing a brick, wielding a club, putting the boot in, or spraying graffiti on walls with a can of
aerosol paint. Whilst noting that clearly not all vandals
are adolescents Cohen (1968) has written that 'studies in
the East End of London indicate that most vandalism occurs

at a younger age in the life cycle than the peak age for
property offences (at that time 14) but some also occurs in
the context of general rowdyism offences in late adolescence.'

Some areas are more prone to vandalism than others.
One explanation for this is that the physical design of a
neighbourhood influences local crime rates. Newman
(1972) looked at the relationship between housing design,
the characteristics of the residents and crime rates. He
argued that although architecture does not have a direct
causal effect on social interaction it does influence those
interactions. He found that crime is more likely to occur
where, for instance, the entrance to flats in a high rise
building is not marked off by steps or a wall as private
space (what he calls 'territoriality') but remains as public
territory where anyone feels free to enter. If this public
space is then hidden from the scrutiny or residents (which
he terms 'natural surveillance'), because it is not overlooked by windows or balconies, it is a space where crime
such as vandalism or mugging is unlikely to be detected and
unlikely to be deterred.

Newman associates crime and trouble with opportunity.
He sees the physical design of an area influencing the
opportunity for trouble to occur. His solution is to produce housing designs which allow for more effective policing of neighbourhoods. What Newman to a large extent
ignores is that trouble may occur as adolescents satisfy
quite understandable needs for fun and excitement in an environment which is drab and monotonous. This may be an
environment which provides little play space or else provides play space which is too public and too uniform, such
as the open spaces between high rise housing or the concrete courtyards surrounded by terraces of low rise walk-
up flats. This is a particularly limiting environment when
the geographical location of these housing complexes is
remote from centres of commercial entertainment, and is
little provided for locally in terms of pubs, clubs and community meeting places. Remoteness in this context may not
only be measured by physical distance. It is also characterised by the imposition of physical obstacles, such as
railway lines and main roads, and by the social ostracism
of the inhabitants of certain neighbourhoods by those from
other localities who see themselves as more 'respectable'.

This is an argument which is developed by Armstrong and
Wilson (1973a and 1973b) in their study of Easterhouse in

Glasgow and by Gill (1977) in his study of adolescents and
trouble in 'Luke Street', a neighbourhood in Crosby.   They
also emphasise that it is not only opportunity and the satisfaction of quite normal needs which can lead to trouble.
There is a third part of the process of trouble occurring
when behaviour is seen as being beyond a level of community or official tolerance and hence is defined as 'trouble'.
   Gill argues that in 'Luke Street' it was housing policy
that led to a decline in the reputation of the neighbourhood.
Luke Street is an area of pre-war corporation housing
designed for large families.   As new housing estates were
built in other areas the older properties of Luke Street
were less desirable with the result that those families already in difficulties with rent arrears, and who were seen
as 'bad' or 'rough' tenants, were housed in Luke Street
(Gill, 1974).   These were often large families with many
children who were experiencing multiple problems and
stresses, especially of finance, and who had little choice
in the housing market.   These families grew up together
and as the children got older there were a number who were
involved in delinquency.   The reputation of Luke Street as
an area of delinquency and trouble was increased by
heightened press coverage of incidents in Luke Street and
by increased policing of the area.   The adolescents came
to see themselves as tough, saw trouble as an avenue for
acceptance among peers, and hence lived up to the reputation of their neighbourhood.   This issue of neighbourhood
reputation and tradition and choice in the housing market is
also related to delinquency by many other studies over
many years:

> Delinquency has become almost a social tradition (in some
> neighbourhoods) and it is only very few youngsters who
> are able to grow up in these areas without at some time
> or other committing illegal acts (Mays, 1954, p. 147).

> one's bargaining power and individual preference in the
> housing market may get one into or out of certain areas;
> ... being in those areas may have very important effects
> on behaviour.   On the present evidence of the Sheffield
> study, the housing market is in the long run much more
> important in differences in crime and offender rates in
> urban areas than either architectural design or police
> patrolling (Bottoms, 1976, p. 6).

Parker (1974), in his participant observation study of
adolescents from a tenement block in Liverpool, also

stresses the impact on young people of living in an area
'with a reputation'. This reputation is accepted by the
adolescents in their confrontations with those outside their
closely defined neighbourhood and they live up to the reputation within their peer groups through a focus on daring
and illegal activities. To a large extent local adults seem
to enter the picture painted by Parker and by Gill as passive observers or as latent sympathisers with much of the
adolescent's behaviour. It seems that in some neighbourhoods unless adults take a firm stand in closely supervising
and controlling the activities of young people it is going to
be very difficult for the young person to stay out of trouble.
When an area has a reputation for trouble and when the
local concerns of the peer group are excitement and fun,
possibly through petty delinquency, then the adolescent on
the street with his friends is likely to be experienced as,
and to be, troublesome. Wilson (1974 and 1978), in her
study of children from large families in an urban environment, found that one of the main characteristics which distinguished those adolescents who did not get into trouble
from those adolescents who were in trouble was the greater
extent to which they were 'chaperoned' by parents. This
characteristic was more important in stopping adolescents
from being involved in delinquency than was a happy home
environment or shared interests and activities between
children and parents.

The importance of adult supervision and surveillance in
curtailing the activities of some adolescents is also
stressed in a Home Office study of vandalism (Marshall,
1976). It concluded that the 'potential for normal social
control within a community is severely restricted if larger-
than-average families are concentrated together thus causing an unmanageably high ratio of children to adults'. The
study also found that areas where there were few opportunities for natural surveillance, or continuing adult scrutiny,
were more vulnerable to vandalism, even though these areas
did not necessarily have a high ratio of children to adults.
It seems, therefore, that a combination of housing design
and of housing policy can lead to some areas experiencing
more trouble, and that this can be related to the physical
difficulties the adults in these areas have in supervising
children and adolescents.

'NEIGHBOURHOOD' AND SOCIAL WORK

So far this paper has discussed how the neighbourhood is of importance to adolescents both as a part of their social development and as a potential element in predisposing some adolescents towards trouble. It remains to discuss how the concept of 'neighbourhood' is of importance to social work philosophy and how this philosophy can be translated into practice in working with adolescents.

'Neighbourhood' and 'community' are often used as synonymous or, at least, closely related terms in social work. During the 1960s and 1970s community work and neighbourhood work have become vogue approaches to social problems. In relation to adolescents the social work/delinquency white papers and the youth service reports of the 1960s, the movement within the education services towards community education, community schools and curriculum development studies with a community focus are all characteristic of the popularising of a community perspective on social problems and issues. Community work received a particular impetus in the context of social work through the Seebohm Report and the report of a Gulbenkian working party.

When we talk about 'community' in the context of social work there seems to be three elements in our conceptualisation (see Dennis, 1958; Plant, 1974; Benson, 1976). First we have some conceptualisation of the size of the social unit we are calling 'a community' and of the number of people who are involved in this unit. We might also have some picture of the geographical location and spread of this unit. This is primarily a physically determined concept of 'community'. Second we have some concept of the social structure of a community – its system of rules and relationships. These are seen to be largely determined by the culture which characterises, signifies and reinforces this system of social interaction. A corollary of this cultural dimension is that the community will have means, both formal and informal, of maintaining its rules and relationships. A third element in our conceptualisation of community is primarily a qualitative evaluation. The evaluative continuum has at one extreme the extended caring and sharing social unit which is largely self-supporting, self-contained and self-policing. At the other extreme of this continuum is the anomic impersonal conglomeration of isolated individuals and families whose interaction is limited to material rather than social or emotional goals.

It is possible to identify at least four advantages of working with adolescents in a neighbourhood context. First,
working with a neighbourhood approach may make more
sense and be more acceptable to the adolescents. If, as
has been suggested above, the neighbourhood is of particular importance to the adolescent's everyday life, and if it
is one of the possible factors predisposing him towards
trouble, then it makes sense to take into account and to work
with his life in his neighbourhood. It is accepted by social
workers and magistrates that neighbourhood attitudes and a
lack of neighbourhood facilities are important factors in the
causation of delinquency (Jones and Kerslake, 1979).
Adolescents in trouble and their parents also stress the
impact of the neighbourhood in the causation of delinquency.
They see the usefulness of much social work as supervising
adolescents while the adolescents take part in normal activities (Jones, 1979). This stops the young people being
bored and also prevents them from roaming the streets,
where they are seen to be at risk of getting into further
trouble. If one of the principles of social work is to 'start
where the client is' and to 'work with his understanding'
then a neighbourhood work approach with adolescents in
trouble is indicated.
    A second advantage of neighbourhood work is that it
focuses on the context in which problems may occur for the
client. There is then the opportunity to increase his
ability to cope with life in his neighbourhood without getting into difficulties. Facing issues of peer group pressures and a limiting environment with the adolescent may
allow one to suggest and rehearse alternative responses to
these pressures, and alternative activities and avenues to
make the environment less limiting. Social workers have
frequently failed to attempt to tackle these issues (Davies,
1973). If one of the aims of social work is to increase the
problem-solving abilities of clients then facing possible
problems together with them is an appropriate approach.
    A third advantage of neighbourhood work is that not only
may it increase the problem-solving capacity of clients, but
it may also create fewer problems for the client in itself.
Recently social work has been accused of hindering rather
than helping those in difficulties (Brandon, 1976). The
accusation is that social work creates and encourages
dependency in those it is trying to help whilst at the same
time stigmatising and ostracising them from the wider community. A social work approach which attempts to provide

a universal rather than a selective stigmatising service reduces the danger of heightening a client's dependency or
deviance. Working with adolescents in trouble, with their
friends, in their neighbourhood, is less likely to single out
and identify some individuals as deviant. It may also possibly allow one to work more comprehensively, and to get
involved before trouble occurs, with others who may be 'at
risk'. Therefore a neighbourhood approach moves us
towards the preventative goal of social work whilst possibly
also reducing the likelihood of social work 'hindering'
clients.

A final advantage of neighbourhood work is that it may
mobilise more resources for the client's benefit. Whilst
social work assistance remains purely an agency duty and
service, the resources which are likely to be made available to distressed, disturbed, deprived and delinquent
adolescents will remain very limited. Social work, or at
least social service provision, may have proliferated over
recent years but the resources social workers have available within their agencies remain small compared to the
need identified. A further approach is to look towards
community resources and also to foster community responsibility for those in need.

The use of community resources is discussed below but
there are particular problems to increasing community responsibility for adolescents. Adolescents are often annoying and confrontational in their behaviour and this does not
increase sympathy for them. Indeed there is often a low
level of tolerance for boisterous young people who play out
on the street. Adolescents do not portray the same picture
of vulnerability or need as young children or the elderly.
For instance, Pearson (1978), in a study of community attitudes in Bradford, found that adolescents were aware of,
and sympathetic to, the problems faced by the elderly in the
community. The elderly, however, saw the adolescents as
a problem, rather than as having problems, although the
adolescents identified many difficulties which they themselves also experienced in the neighbourhood. It seems
that young people per se are often seen as a problem, regardless of their actual behaviour.

Adolescents also often appear not so receptive of help.
The result is that they may be isolated within their neighbourhood or they may be rejected by it. It is the tackling
of this issue which moves us some way towards the further-
ance of the caring and sharing community even if the ultimate
utopia is never to be reached.

WORKING IN THE NEIGHBOURHOOD

But how does one work with adolescents within the neighbourhood? What resources can the neighbourhood offer?
One neighbourhood resource is the indigenous population.
Adults living within a neighbourhood possess a range of
skills and interests which it may be possible to make available to adolescents. Indeed many local people may already
be helping young people by running youth clubs and football
teams and by just being available to talk with young people
about hobbies and, possibly, worries. One of the possible
benefits of encouraging local people to give time and to make
a commitment to the young people around them may be that
the adults will be more readily accessible to the adolescents. They will also probably be available over a longer
period of time than many professionals. Social workers
tend to live away from the neighbourhoods where their young
clients live and they also frequently change jobs in the
search for further stimulation and promotion. These
trends reduce the accessibility and continuity of the service which social workers offer to young people

Working with the indigenous population

But how does one set about identifying local people who may
be willing to help adolescents? One method is to consider
those with whom one, as a social worker, already has contact within a neighbourhood. These might be the parents
of adolescents who are in trouble or other clients who are
known in the locality. The father of one adolescent, who
was being supervised by a social worker, had an interest in
football. His son and his son's friends also had this interest but father and son never actively shared the interest
together. The social worker arranged for a youth club to
select a football team to play a team composed of his adolescent client and the client's friends. The client's father
was persuaded to come to the match and to coach his son's
team. The outcome was that the father continued to coach
the team and they applied to join a local junior soccer
league. The social worker continued to show an interest
in the team and to spectate occasionally at matches. However, it was left to the father, and some other parents, to
organise and manage the team. The result was that a group
of over ten boys were involved in a regular activity where

they received interest, encouragement and supervision from adults whilst having fun. This is not an uncommon experience. For instance, a conference report on intermediate treatment states that:

A youth worker vividly described the two hundred football teams who play on Hackney Marshes on a Saturday morning; two thousand lads playing football, one hundred referees, two hundred managers and trainers, parents, friends, supporters and some two hundred mums washing the kits after every match (Pagan, 1978).

A second example of mobilising local adults to help young people is drawn from the work of the Bath Community Child Care Project (see Fry, 1978). This project is located on a housing estate which has a higher incidence of delinquent young people than other areas of the city. The project combines the approaches of casework, groupwork and community work as the two full-time workers provide a service to young people on the estate. Both the workers live in the neighbourhood where they work. Initially all the homes in the area were approached by the workers. This allowed the workers to discuss the project with local people, and it also helped them to identify possible resource people in the neighbourhood who were sympathetic to the aims of the project and might be willing to offer assistance.

One of the programmes which has developed within this project is a summer play scheme for children and young people on the estate. During the school holidays there is a programme of playgroups, youth clubs, and of small group work with adolescents in trouble. This programme catered for over eighty children and young people during the summer of 1977. To manage a programme of this size required more than two workers, and a 'team' of local adults was recruited. They were paid on a sessional basis and helped to stimulate and supervise the playgroups and youth clubs. The helpers included local parents, the shopkeeper, and some of the older adolescents. It is now planned that the summer play scheme will be an annual event. Certainly during the year following the first play scheme there have been spin-offs such as a Christmas party for the children which parents helped to organise, and parents-children cricket and football matches.

A third way of recruiting local volunteers to help young people is to advertise. Advertising might include formal advertisements in local newspapers. Other, and possibly more fruitful, forms are to have feature articles in the

local press about the work of existing volunteers or to
talk to local community associations and community groups.
One intermediate treatment programme which ran for three
years, and catered during that time for over fifty adolescents, primarily involved only two social workers. The
remaining adult supervision of the programme was provided
by ten volunteers, some of whom approached the social services department offering help following an extensive report
in the local press about the work of volunteers.

An additional gain with several of these volunteers was
that they lived on the same estates and in the same streets
as the adolescents with whom they worked. These adolescents frequently called on the volunteers outside the organised events within the intermediate treatment programme.
They took the volunteer's dog for a walk, played cards with
him, went swimming with the volunteer's family, and helped
wash the volunteer's car. They shared everyday life experiences with the volunteers. The adolescents had found
some adults who lived near them with whom they could share
activities, spend time and talk about current personal
issues.

A problem for the volunteers was to control the demands
the adolescents made on them. The volunteers required
support and assistance in clarifying their role and this was
offered through group discussions and through individual
contact between the social workers and the volunteers.
Hence although the volunteers greatly enriched the service
provided to the adolescents, and in some cases to other
members of the adolescent's family as well, it is salutory
to remember that:

> Many social workers have recognised – most notably in
> the probation service – that volunteers do not save time,
> they take time; to recruit, to train, to organise and to
> supervise; and although they can be a valuable additional
> resource, it is short sighted to imagine that they will not
> make demands on the existing structure (Davies, 1977,
> p. 5).

This quotation is taken from a book which discusses the
work of volunteers with ESN school leavers and their families. Another account of a project with adolescents in the
community which was largely staffed by volunteers is the
Wincroft Youth Project (Smith et al., 1972). However in
both of these projects the volunteers did not necessarily
live in the same neighbourhoods as the adolescents with
whom they were working. An account of using local adults

to work with adolescents is provided by Thorpe in his
account of 'multi-dimensional social work methods' in
Nottingham (9172). Parents and neighbours were encouraged to run activities for young people in an area which had
few recreational, social or entertainment facilities but had
a high incidence of juvenile delinquents. The local Tenants
and Residents Association also became involved in helping
young people. This suggests that existing community
groups, such as neighbourhood associations, tenants
groups, and community councils may be well located and
willing to help to provide facilities for young people, although Robins and Cohen (1978) would question this. They
found a good deal of conflict between the adolescents they
were assisting and local formal community groups.

Working with natural friendship groups

One form of neighbourhood group which has often been neglected by social workers is the natural friendship group of
adolescents. Social work agencies usually structure their
work into caseloads where workers work with 'cases' or
possibly groups of cases. There is an inbuilt difficulty in
locating the client in his everyday social environment and
working with him in this environment (see Chapter three).
This may entail working with him and his friends together.
A result of this is likely to be additional work for the social
worker, who may find that he is getting involved with other
adolescents and their families who never appear on his
workload returns and who are not considered when work is
being allocated:

> Because of the whole system of caseloads, of files, of
> supervision of work, and of allocation of resources, many
> chances of helping groups of people to act more effective-
> ly together, and to press for better conditions, go
> wasted, while social workers seek unavailingly to lure
> individuals, and especially adolescents, away from
> groups which might more profitably be helped, as groups,
> to engage in more satisfying and constructive activities,
> or be provided with better facilities in which to interact
> together (Jordan, 1972, p. 139).

To a large extent working with natural friendship groups
remains the role of the youth service, but social workers
are also entering this field. They may be working with a
client and a few of his friends whilst carrying a tradition-

ally structured caseload (Emerson et al., 1977). In other
examples social workers have been employed as detached
youth workers where:

> the method of work is to move into the neighbourhoods
> and establish contact with young people where they are,
> rather than expecting them to move towards the worker or
> any building. It is argued that this approach leaves the
> control of the contact very much in the young person's
> hands, and she can determine the speed at which the con-
> tact develops and the way in which it is used (Marchant
> and Smith, 1977, p. 11).

Detached youth workers focus their work on 'unattached'
young people. These are young people who have little involvement with existing youth facilities and whose life is
characterised by drifting. This drifting could signify existing personal difficulties and it could also lead them into
further trouble such as delinquency, drug abuse, homeless-
ness or promiscuity. These young people make little use
of conventional youth service provision, may well be unemployed or (if younger) truanting, and are often the clients of
social workers. A service which 'reaches out' to these
young people on terms acceptable to them falls between the
responsibility of the youth service and the social services
and probation services. It might be appropriate for detached youth work projects in a neighbourhood to be jointly
funded by education departments and by social service
departments. This would help to move this form of work
with young people from its present experimental status into
a more established, more continuous provision. Detached
youth work has the advantage of working with the adolescent
at his pace. It provides a more locally accessible service
which is also less formal. A similar service may be
offered to adolescents through drop-in counselling centres,
but these are not so often neighbourhood based but cover a
larger catchment area (see, for instance, Humphries,
1977, and Tomkins, 1978).

Using local facilities

Further possible neighbourhood resources for young
people, in addition to the people who live or work in the
neighbourhood with them, are the organised amenities and
the physical environment of the locality. Within most
neighbourhoods there are likely to be youth clubs, church

halls and schools. It may be that the adolescent is already using these facilities. For instance, a survey in
1969 found that 72 per cent of boys and 58 per cent of girls
were attached to some form of club and that 93 per cent
had been involved with a club at some time (OPCS, 1969).
However, research on adolescents and young people in contact with social workers (Jones, 1979) and probation officers (Davies, 1969) has found that they tend not to use youth
clubs regularly. If they attend at all their attendance is
very sporadic. For some of these adolescents it may well
be that youth clubs would have great difficulty in containing
their disruptive behaviour. Accounts of particularly challenging and destructive behaviour are to be found in many
accounts of youth work with previously unattached young
people (Spencer, 1964; Goetschius and Tash, 1967; Daniel
and McGuire, 1972).

But for some young people it is not their confrontational
behaviour which excludes them from using local amenities.
It is rather their lack of confidence which results in a
passivity and an unwillingness to risk unknown experiences
and to cross new thresholds. There is a role for the
social worker to work at increasing the adolescent's confidence and to nurture him with the eventual aim of introduc-
ing him to, and supporting him through, membership and
participation in local clubs and organised activities. One
10-year-old boy, for instance, was isolated within his age
group and in his class at school. Whilst encouraging the
parents to be more supportive of their very insecure son
the social worker also persuaded the boy to attend a small
intermediate treatment group with him. When the boy first
attended he was so frightened that he was physically sick.
Over a period of months, however, the boy's confidence increased and he was helped to join the Cubs. When he
moved to a secondary school there was an initial decline
again in his confidence, but he soon became an enthusiastic
member of the school's chess club and of an extra curricular
school gymnastic club. He also became a regular attender
of a local church's youth club.

A form of neighbourhood facility which is very much related to the work of social workers but is often not seen as a
neighbourhood resource is the residential establishment.
One of the confusions inherent in the changing terminology
of child care and juvenile corrections is the use of the term
'community home' to replace what were previously called
'approved schools' and 'children's homes' (see Chapter

eight).   What is meant by a 'community home'?   Is it a home
which is run as a community, a home which is a part of a
community, or is it just a home for those excluded from the
community?   Many community homes are now being integrated much more fully into the life of the neighbourhood where
they are located.   This has been true for a long time for
smaller family group homes, but some of the conglomera-
tions of cottage homes and homes with education on the premises were detached from the life of the community around
them.   However residential social workers have much to
offer the adolescents in their neighbourhood in terms of
interest and stimulation.

   It has also been suggested that there is much to be gained
from placing many adolescents who are received into care
in placements which allow them to remain in close contact
with their family and friends.   It is likely that they will
ultimately return to live in their own neighbourhood again
anyway and hence they need to be helped to cope with,
rather than being separated from, the problems they face at
home.   Tutt has argued for the development of community
homes which serve a small locality.   They would provide
accommodation not just for younger children and adolescents
but also for the elderly and handicapped who need residential care.   They would also work with others in the adolescent's everyday environment.   A local establishment of this
type which was 'firmly based within the community, offering
a service to the child's family, friends and school, could
really begin to call itself a community home' (Tutt, 1974,
p. 206).

   Jordan (1972) has also discussed the advantages of neighbourhood-based care for those adolescents who cannot live
at home.   He suggests the use of local people, who may already be within the network of contacts and friends of the
adolescent, as a possible resource when an adolescent is
rejected by his immediate family.   Placing the adolescent
with people he already knows, in an environment with which
he is already familiar, may be less traumatic to him at what
is already a time of personal crisis.   An account of a community home which is catering for local children, and is integrated into the life of its neighbourhood, is offered by
Hudson (1978).   Recollections of other experiences where
children's homes have provided day care for local children
during holidays, or allowed space to be used for a youth
club, emphasise the practicability and benefits of residential establishments and residential social workers being
seen as a neighbourhood resource.

Involving the adolescent in the neighbourhood

So far the discussion on working with adolescents within the neighbourhood has focused on adolescents taking from, and using, neighbourhood resources. Other approaches include working with the adolescent's experience and awareness of his neighbourhood, and also getting adolescents to provide a community service.

Adolescents, especially adolescents in trouble, know that their presence in the neighbourhood is often unwelcomed by many people. Neighbours complain about the noise that they make, and parents of other children try to prevent their children from associating with troublesome teenagers. Shopkeepers watch what they perceive as these potential shoplifters with an eagle eye. They are discouraged from playing and meeting in the playgrounds for younger children and in the pubs and clubs aimed at an adult market. Yet this is still the locality where the adolescent rendezvous with his friends and where he has his established haunts. But the adolescent may still be unaware of much that happens in his neighbourhood. He can be an outsider even within his own locality.

Many aspects and parts of the neighbourhood will be out-of-bounds to the adolescent. His impression of his locality may be only a barely clad skeleton of what is happening around him. Exclusion from what is happening around him is unlikely to lead to an increased commitment to the fabric and life of his immediate environment. In an attempt to compensate for these limiting experiences, visits to local services, such as the fire station and the police station, and to local factories and industries, take the adolescent from the position of the unknowing outsider, or the uninformed observer, towards a position of increased knowledge about, and involvement in, the everyday life of his locality.

This involvement in, and commitment to, the wider aspects of life in the neighbourhood may also be furthered by the adolescents offering a service to his community:

Service to the community provides the opportunity to change the role of the young person from that of 'receiver' to 'giver' and helper, thus offering a counterbalance to the traditional role the young person with difficulties often finds himself in, as the recipient of advice and treatment. The opportunity to help others not only enables the young person to develop his talents and skills in the service of others and to appreciate their needs, but encourages him

to realise his own worth. A contribution made to the
community may also encourage integration into it, perhaps
helped by contact with many different sections of the community (Personal Social Services Council, 1977, p. 57).
Recent examples of adolescents and young people in
trouble providing a community service for others include
the Hammersmith Teenage Project, with its emphasis on
'new careers' where 'young people who have themselves
been in trouble with the law are employed to help teenagers
to keep out of trouble' (Whitlam, 1977). Another example
is the Lambeth Community Service Volunteers Scheme,
where adolescents are involved in community service during
the day as an alternative to residential care (Knight, 1977).
In the example discussed earlier of the intermediate treatment programme which was run mainly by volunteers, one of
the volunteers was a 19-year-old who had himself recently
spent four years in various community homes and who had
himself been involved in delinquency.

DIFFICULTIES AND CONSTRAINTS

One of the advantages of involving adolescents in community
service activities is that it may help to modify the way in
which the community sees adolescents who have been difficult. Rather than having a holistic perception of them as
'bad', their involvement in community service may present
a picture of these adolescents which also shows them to be
capable of constructive and co-operative activity. However a major constraint within the neighbourhood approach
is that the tiresome, trying and sometimes traumatic behaviour of some adolescents will outstrip community tolerance.
A tension is always likely to exist between challenging
adolescents and the adults they confront. In commenting
on work with one particularly difficult group of young
people, Spencer states that:
  Groupwork among adolescents as disturbed as the Es-
  pressos, and with personal histories like theirs, must
  always be frightening and perplexing to any neighbourhood, particularly a somewhat insecure new estate. It
  is easier to let the individuals drift and to let the social
  services and police pick up the consequences in personal
  and family breakdown and delinquency at once or later
  (Spencer, 1964, pp. 162-3).
But possibly this tension between adults and adolescents

within a neighbourhood can to some extent be diffused by
making the adolescents and adults more considerately aware
of, and concerned about, each other. This might be achieved by some of the forms of adult-adolescent contact suggested above as appropriate ways of working within the neighbourhood. However it has to be accepted, and it is appropriate, that some behaviours can not be tolerated within a
community and that some small number of adolescents will
have to be removed from their immediate community.

Yet it is not only the community that imposes constraints
on the use of a neighbourhood approach with difficult adolescents. It has already been commented that the way in
which many social work agencies organise their work loads
may inhibit the use of a neighbourhood approach. A neighbourhood approach with adolescents in trouble is facilitated
by multi-disciplinary teams organised on a patch system.
The National Children's Bureau study (Leissner et al.,
1977) of how family advice centres provided a service to
young people portrays this approach in action. But even if
one's own agency encourages a neighbourhood approach
other agencies may disapprove:

In all the projects, intensive work with the 'hard core'
youngsters caused problems with regard to the relations
with other agencies. Resentment of accepting attitudes
towards delinquents and habitual truants and lack of
understanding of the objectives of the project was (with
some notable exceptions) most pronounced in relations
with the police and schools (Leissner et al., 1977, p. 24).

However, on the same page, there is a quote from a police-
man who helped build an adventure playground with one of
the projects. He said that 'it must stare most of my colleagues in the face that the youth workers' influence has
led to a reduction in delinquency in the area.... It is surprising how much constructive activity has been initiated by
kids who, three years ago, seemed hell bent on trouble.'
This again suggests that co-operative contact between local
adolescents and adults can change the picture and stereotype which is held of the adolescent.

A final constraint to the neighbourhood approach may be
the constraints we each impose for ourselves. Social
workers have been described as 'commuter do-gooders' and
as 'external caretakers'. We live away from the neighbourhoods where we work and where the adolescents are
'in action'. This may to some extent be necessary for our
own survival. Accounts of detached youth workers living

in the areas where they work show how stressful can be the
continual accessibility to them by the young people with
whom they are working (see, for instance, Collins, 1977).
A neighbourhood approach does not necessarily mean that
one needs to live in the neighbourhood where one is working, but certainly being a resident of the neighbourhood
takes one's work on to a different level of intensity and
involvement.

CONCLUDING COMMENT

This paper has argued that the neighbourhood is of much
importance to adolescents, and that in working with adolescents in trouble there is a great deal to be gained by working with them in the context of their neighbourhood. Counselling and groupwork with difficult and deprived young
people would be enriched by being integrated into their
everyday environment. The penultimate chapter in this
book suggests that adolescents may be particularly challenging clients for the social worker. This chapter challenges some of the traditional ways we have developed for
working with these adolescents. By using a neighbourhood
perspective to look again at our established ways of working
with young people we may be able to make our work more
relevant to them.

Chapter eight

Residential care and adolescents

John Burns, William Gregory
and Graham Templeman

/This chapter explores some issues which arise in providing residential care for adolescents. It discusses in some detail the model of residential work as practised in one community home with education, and describes some of the techniques used in this setting. The reasons for admission into care, and the varying perceptions of this care, are discussed, and the chapter also describes some of the stresses experienced by residential social workers. It needs to be emphasised that although this chapter focuses on caring for adolescents who are delinquent, a large number of the adolescents in residential care are neither delinquent nor especially difficult./

PERCEPTIONS AND EXPECTATIONS OF COMMUNITY HOMES

All homes for children and young people within the context of our official arrangements for social services are set up within the Community Homes System. The term 'Community Home' bears examination. Presumably recent changes in the law brought about a change in name from 'Children's Home' to 'Community Home' for a specific purpose, but what was that purpose? Clearly any community home must have a community of people within it; thus the children with the staff of the home must be a community. Is this what the term 'Community Home' means? Does it, perhaps, mean something slightly different? Is it a community of children who live in that particular home, i.e. to the exclusion of the staff who work there? Again, is the concept a different one; is it the concept of a home which is part of the commu-

nity in which it is set?   Or is it a home for children run on
behalf of the community - community being defined as that
local part of society which is responsible for its running?
    The Children and Young Persons Act 1969 set up the
regional-based Public System of Community Homes.   Wales
is one region and England is divided into eleven regions.
All establishments providing residential care for children
and run or controlled by local authorities are included in
the system.   Additionally some places owned and run by
voluntary agencies have a local authority component in
their management and are also within the system.   Thus,
the system includes nurseries, small family group homes,
other children's homes of varying sizes, reception centres,
and observation and assessment centres, hostels, former
remand homes and former approved schools.   The latter
usually provide education on the premises but the others do
not, and the units vary in size and in the facilities which
they can offer.   Some have room for only very small num-
bers of children whilst others can cater for perhaps 40.
Most accept boys and girls; others are single sex establishments.   The former approved schools are often complex
establishments catering for perhaps up to 100 children and
have a wide range of facilities and staff of many disciplines.
These differences compound the confusion inherent in the
generic title 'Community Home'.   They also limit and to
some extent control what social and other work can be
offered to their residents.   The image of each home as perceived by the local community, the local authority, the
local authority social services managers, the children and
their parents, and others including members of the police
and legal professions, affects their functioning.
    Because the various agencies and parts of society have
different views about a community home they also have differing expectations about the results which a community
home might achieve.   These very expectations will affect
the possible treatment methods as compared with the therapeutic, helping ideals which those responsible and working
within the home might themselves have.   Thus, society may
well expect that a young car thief shall be committed to a
residential institution and be treated so that he no longer
takes and drives away cars.   The residential institution
chosen by society as its therapeutic instrument can possibly
be totally inhibited in achieving that objective simply because the society will not allow the home to operate in the
way in which it needs to do if society's stated expectations

are to be fulfilled.   One of the clearest examples of this is
when a young person has been committed to residential care
because of sexually deviant behaviour.   Often a necessary
component of the treatment is to allow the young person to
be treated by and come into close contact with people of the
opposite sex.   This can be seen as threatening by the outside community.   As a result direct or indirect action can
be taken by that community to prevent the residential establishment acting in a way which the professional workers see
as essential to the young person's sexual health.

This leads on to consideration of another facet of the community's expectations about residential care.   Residential
care is often expected to cure presenting behaviour.   The
task willed upon residential care is to eradicate the behaviour which society sees as obnoxious.   Sometimes this can
be done but the elimination of such behaviour by no means
guarantees that all the child's undesirable behaviour will be
eradicated nor does it ensure that any substituted behaviour
will be acceptable.   A classic case of this kind of difficulty
was encountered in the early days of long-stay secure
establishments within the approved school system.   One of
the prime reasons for setting up such establishments was to
prevent young people who had persistently absconded from
continuing to do so.   It was not recognised, however, that
often continued absconding was an expression by the individual of panic and of an inability to face his own problems.
Consequently, when these young people were put into a
secure setting and could no longer run away from the
actuality of their own problems they often became aggressive, and often this aggression was directed towards the
staff.   This behaviour then led to criticism of the staff, as
the staff were seen as carrying out their duties incorrectly
because these panic-stricken children had no previous history of violence towards staff in the (open) approved schools
in which they had previously been resident.

Whatever a community home actually is many people and
many agencies will hold varying beliefs about it, whilst it
also will have views of the various agencies and people
outside itself.   These relationships can be extremely com-
plicated and it may be that the staff of the home will define
the difficult behaviour of the adolescent as having its roots
in the family or in the community (see Walter, 1978).   Thus
work with the family, field workers and schools are essential functions of the residential task.

AIMS AND USES OF RESIDENTIAL CARE

Residential care may be separated into two main areas.
The first we will call positive residential care: it is that
kind of residential care chosen for what it has to offer a
particular client. It is deliberately chosen because it has
advantages over other forms of care. They may be that
the residential setting gives opportunities to intervene
which would not otherwise exist, or that the intervention
can be more frequent more intensive and in a 'safer' and
more controlled setting. Thus the client's emotional responses can be ventilated and explored in the safety that
does not normally exist in the community and can be tolerated over longer periods.

Other residential care can be called passive. Some
young people need to be protected from the stresses of
family life and of the community, or perhaps from the anger
of society. This is particularly so for some young people
whose offences or behaviour society sees as particularly
offensive or damaging. Obvious examples are the taking of
life and patterns of severely deviant sexual behaviour.
However, the behaviour of children who need protection is
not necessarily extraordinary; a community can become extremely angry about a small group of young people commit-
ting relatively minor offences. Sometimes the demands are
made that the young people should be 'sent away' and 'locked
up'. If the law and its administration appears weak such
demands can be more vociferous: it is perhaps no accident
that it is under the liberal 1969 Act that we are providing
more secure places for juveniles in the child care system.

It needs to be remembered that how a young person be-
haves causes variable responses from adults including parents, adults in authority and the forces of law and order
(Woolf, 1967). Of three children acting similarly one will
be treated as delinquent, another as in need of treatment,
and the third may be ignored altogether. This kind of
double standard may help explain the slowness in the development of intermediate treatment and the increase in commit-
tals to Detention Centres and to Borstal Training. Society
demands punishment for those it perceives as delinquents
but sees the measures available under the 1969 Act as
treatment.

It is quite clear that for any particular group of young
people the positive and passive aspects of residential care
are not necessarily discrete but often overlap. The ways

in which adolescents are referred for residential care and the stated reasons for the referrals tell us something about the perceived objectives of residential care. Most adolescents come into residential care because they are perceived by social workers and others as young people with problems, but society sees them as young people who are difficult to manage, i.e. that they are difficult for adults to manage. This causes a demand for the use of residential care methods rather than community-based methods. Society feels more comfortable if the young people it sees as threatening are dealt with in a way it sees as positive. In relation to the use of secure accommodation Hoghughi (1978a) calls attention to public attitudes expressed to and by the House of Commons Expenditure Committee Report (1975). He points out that the assertion of social control is seen as a major element in all forms of social intervention: such assertion reduces the feeling of impotence on the part of social agencies and increases their peace of mind. Burns (1977) postulated that unease on the part of the police about the effectiveness of the 1969 Act caused them to report more delinquents than they had done previously. Such pressures can cause the admission to residential care of some adolescents who have no positive need of treatment and thus from the social work perspective this kind of action is negative. However, negative reasons for the use of residential care do not negate its positive potential, for the residential workers can assist the adolescent to progress towards maturity by enriching his developmental experiences. This is what the residential social workers perceive to be their prime task no matter for what reasons or by what process the adolescent entered residential care.

However, Utting (1977), in discussing the purpose and values of residential care, has stated that changes are needed, generally in the direction of providing for the more disturbed and more difficult people. The Children and Young Persons Act 1969 was based on this concept, expecting intermediate treatment to keep the lesser disturbed and difficult in the community, and Rutherford (1977) has shown how there is some attempt in the USA to cut back on the extent of official intervention in the lives of young offenders, based on the premise that such intervention is counter-productive. There has been much discussion on the need to replace residential care by means based upon the community. Whatever the extent of the success of such approaches no doubt residential care will remain, and

Burns (1977) suggested that a continuum of care, treatment
and control is necessary for the benefit of young people
themselves.

RESIDENTIAL CARE AND RESIDENTIAL SOCIAL WORK

It is usual to speak of residential care and of residential
care workers. In many ways this appears to enshrine an
outmoded concept. Often in residential institutions, particularly those concerned with adolescents, the young
people are resident but the staff are not. That tells us
something of the way in which the objectives of residential
care are now pursued and the way in which they differ from
those previously thought to be of prime importance.
Until comparatively recently residential care was the
means by which a single straightforward theme was pursued;
the aim of providing a substitute home by using paid surrogate parents operating in a residential setting. This is
still reflected in much residential child care today, for example, by the use of such terms as 'housemother' and
'housefather'. Such apparently simple aims are still pursued in some residential settings; however it is now generally assumed that children needing only a substitute home
should be in foster homes or adoptive homes. There can
be no simple and clear-cut demarcation between children
who should and should not be in residential care. Some
children need substitute parenting but cannot accept the
closeness of relationships in a family and consequently need
alternative arrangements. Others need protection: an
example is quoted later in this chapter. Jones (1979)
speaks of such needs when discussing the residential community as a setting for social work.
We suggest, like Allen (1977), that the overall objectives
of residential social work must be those of social work
itself pursued by way of the special factors which the residential situation adds. Put simply, the residential setting
allows more control of the total environment and more
opportunity to use social work, and other techniques, and
to use them more effectively. Hence the worker is normally one of a team that is in constant contact with the client.
It should be noted, therefore, that residential care is not
necessarily confined to residential social work. Payne
(1977) suggested that many children are so damaged or disruptive that they can be helped only within a residential

setting with the help they need given them not only by social
work but by workers of several disciplines. The interaction of multi-disciplinary staff merits considerable
study. In many specialised institutions there is an emphasis on inter-disciplinary working methods in which staffs
of varying disciplines deliberately commit themselves to
step over the boundaries of their own profession and to
allow their fellow team members to step over their boundaries so that there is a merging of the various disciplines.
We will be referring to some of these processes and methods later in the chapter.

We have by inference made reference to some of the methods by which young people are looked after and treated
within residential care. We have seen that compared with
earlier periods there are more complex approaches being
operated at the present time. Most of the methodologies
now being used are based on the premise that it is possible
to discover the causes of the presenting behaviour difficulties and thereby prescribe the treatment which the young
person needs. It also presumes that young people's presenting problems can be treated and that therapeutic
approaches are not only possible but ought to be used.
This postulates that there has been something wrong in the
child's upbringing and that if this can be identified then the
appropriate treatment to remedy the situation can be
applied. As a result approaches based on the idea that
young people also need a disciplined setting have been
attacked as being backward and repressive, whilst by comparison methods which are claimed to be 'therapeutic' are
seen as progressive and good.

However, therapeutic methods are not necessarily seen
by the adolescent to be less punitive than those methods
which professional workers regard as authoritarian and
harsh. Burns (1977) called attention to experiences
suggesting that children would prefer to be sent to a short-
term authoritarian Detention Centre rather than be committed by a court on a potentially long-term order designed to
allow flexible treatment. Young people prefer to know
where they stand: a therapeutic milieu can be experienced
as limbo and therefore be felt to be highly punitive. In
this connection Gill (1974) and Walter (1978) describe institutions which are seen by the staff as providing help but
are often seen by the young people as punitive. It is thus
hardly surprising to find that Martinson (1974), in an examination of the research literature, found that the rehabili-

tative efforts that have been reported so far have had no appreciable effect on recidivism and that there are no significant differences in success rates between community treatment programmes and institutional methods.

It has also rarely been possible to demonstrate by evaluating results scientifically that any one method is more successful than another in any given situation or for a specific group of 'clients' (Clarke and Cornish, 1972 and 1975). However this has not prevented the various protagonists from claiming that their own particular ways were the best. Young people have rarely been asked for their own views, but when this had been done they have shown considerable insight and a very straightforward approach to what they perceive as their particular needs. Thus in the Dartington survey (Millham et al., 1975) of community homes with education (when they were still approved schools) the young people demonstrated that most of all they valued those places and those members of staff who could give them the means to obtain and continue in employment (see also Dunlop, 1974). They viewed employment as the means of obtaining money regularly whilst remaining free of the clutches of the law; they also showed that they did not want money for its own sake but for what it could provide for them.

More recently young people have shown that they are not convinced by people who profess to be acting altruistically by, for example, providing a foster home for a deprived or delinquent child; there is at least some evidence from the young people themselves (Page and Clarke, 1977) that they would prefer a more professional arrangement. This probably applies especially to those young people who have families and homes of their own. These young people may be well aware that their parents and homes do not provide them with the proper ingredients for a progressive development towards adulthood. This does not mean that they are prepared to accept an alternative home. They may, however, be prepared and willing and able to accept help offered by social workers and others operating in a residential setting. Young people like to know, indeed need to know, where they stand in relation to the adults in their life. Those young people seen by society as having problems or as problem young people can often accept assistance but cannot accept the usurping by would-be surrogate parents of their own parents' positions however damaging the parents might be (see also Holman, 1975, for a discussion of this issue in relation to styles of fostering).

ASSESSMENT

Referrals of such young people are frequently problem-centred whilst the work with them needs to be task-centred. So the question arises whether it is practical to 'assess a child' and thereby find 'remedies'. Intense and sophisticated analysis and assessment, with the consequent exposure of the defects and limitations of the child's upbringing and past history, will not necessarily indicate the way in which the young person can be helped. More usually it will show the way in which the child might be managed and might be assisted in some areas. There is considerable doubt that assessment of the child's actual 'being' will give us the clues to the components of therapeutic endeavour upon which we should engage in an attempt to heal the young person. This is not to say that assessment should not be undertaken nor that assessment can never match the young person's needs to a suitable treatment facility. If this is accepted then assessment is not merely useful but an absolute necessity. Assessment is our means whereby the young person can become a known quantity and therefore our passport in our attempts to assist the young person. Assessment must not be seen merely as the gateway to placement in a residential facility.

Assessment, of course, begins when the child first comes to the notice of the authorities, and it is then that the first decision is made regarding the child's future. Treatment also begins at this stage for every action taken by the responsible adult has some effect on the child. The diagnosis must be accurate and rigorous. This assessment need not take place in a residential setting, but sometimes this may prove necessary.

A major part of assessment, whether it be residential or not, must be identifying problems and discovering why these have occurred. This requires the expertise of a range of specialists to gain a reasonably accurate and balanced picture of the child. Within a residential setting, which has a staff comprised of these specialists, it is comparatively easy to do this. These various people work as an inter-disciplinary team so they are able to get a deep understanding of the problem by frequent and regular cross-reference. An important part of gaining an accurate composite picture of the child lies in the individual disciplines being able to view the child from their own specialist angle and draw on, and use, the investigations of the others. It is essential

that such inter-disciplinary teams are responsible for
assessment, whether it is carried out on a day, peripatetic
or residential basis.

There have been many attempts to evaluate the validity of
assessment but this is difficult because the eventual outcome in any individual case is dependent on treatment as
well as the assessment.   Also objective measures of success and failure, such as recidivism rates, are influenced
by many variables, such as policing policy, which are external to the adolescent.   Hoghughi (1978b) states that the
outcome of any assessment can be evaluated in terms of
certain basic criteria.   These include:

Reliability   – the degree to which findings can be trusted
                 regardless of circumstances.

Validity   – the degree to which assessment shows the
                 person as he really is.

Efficiency   – how well the outcome measures up against
                 the expenditure and resources.

Rigour   – the thoroughness of the scrutiny, and
                 organisation of the process of assessment

Relevance   – how much the outcome of assessment throws
                 light on the particular problem.

Utility   – the degree to which assessment can satisfy
                 the purpose for which it was intended.

If our concept of 'positive' residential care is to be realised then a full and detailed assessment is the only way of
ensuring that tasks are identified so the subsequent placement can be task and treatment orientated and not problem-
centred.   The assessment report should be written to reflect strictly the findings of the assessment process, and
never in such a way to make it appear that the subject is a
suitable match to a specific treatment facility.   If these
ideals are met then the real needs that exist can be identified and defects in the existing provision exposed, whilst at
the same time the treatment facility chosen for an adolescent
would be in possession of accurate information which would
enable its staff team to amend its techniques appropriately.
Finding, or attempting to find, an appropriate placement is
a crucial part of assessment.   Sufficient time must be devoted to finding the appropriate facility by a person with
adequate knowledge of the facilities available.   The decision must not be made in terms of the seriousness of the
presenting problem; it must reflect the needs of the individual.   However, occasionally it may be inevitable and
necessary in the case of a child who presents a major threat

to the community, or endangers himself, to override this basic concept.

What happens when no appropriate facility exists or none will accept the child? In some cases it may be possible to prepare the child for future placement by implementing some form of short-term treatment and sometimes this can be done in the assessment centre utilising its specialist resources. In other cases it may be that the necessary provision is not available, or, possibly, that no one knows what should be done for a particular individual. Present knowledge and resources do not resolve all adolescents' problems.

STRUCTURING RESIDENTIAL WORK

As the residential task is so complex one approach is to view it as made up of a number of components. Goals and sub-goals associated with these components and the overall task can be described and methods to attain these goals can be delineated and their use monitored. Most such approaches are based upon behaviour modification theories and an English example is described by Burland and Mather (1978). One approach which allows the use of a variety of methods is the TRACE system (Treatment Recording and Case Evaluation) which was developed in the Adolescent Unit of Whitby Psychiatric Hospital, Ontario, and has since been modified and used in several residential establishments in this country. In brief, the TRACE system consists of:
  (a) goal setting.
  (b) treatment planning,
  (c) evaluation of treatment outcome, and
  (d) recording.
It is essentially a way of structuring a treatment programme and setting it out in the form of specific concrete goals. This is done in such a way that the programme can be evaluated later. This puts far more objectivity and accountability into the work (Tennal School, 1976).

The system starts by assessing and then analysing the child's basic needs and then setting them out in a simple, precise and systematised manner. As adapted there are five basic areas which are examined in depth:
   (i) educational/vocational,
  (ii) physical/medical,
 (iii) personal/psychic,
  (iv) social/behavioural and
   (v) familial/cultural.

Each of these areas is further subdivided into a number of
categories. A programme Summary Sheet is set out which
records the specific programme to be followed for a specified period of time. This is the overall treatment programme which includes the problem areas, the ameliorative
experiences and the goals. Following the completion of
the Summary Sheet the detail is written up on the Service
Method Sheet, clearly stating the first stage towards
achieving each goal; in practice it has been found that six
is the maximum number of goals that can be effectively
worked on simultaneously. Each area is referred to by a
code letter in order that any daily recordings made by staff
(each member of staff must record at least daily) are related to a specific area of the programme. The Daily Record
Sheet for each boy is examined each month together with the
Treatment Programme, and by referring to the code letter
a progress picture in each area is readily available. The
team and the individual member of staff responsible for
each area has to account for any lack of progress at this
stage and each review is recorded. An actual example of
a boy who was placed on a short-term treatment is given
below:

Tony had committed sexual offences against very young
girls in his home, urban area. The local population was
outraged at his conduct. He had been physically threatened, for example, with carving knives. On entry to the
Assessment Centre he presented as a sorrowful, tearful,
anxious, homesick, unkempt and extremely sad boy who,
additionally, was extremely lonely. He was unused to
having friends although he was a friendly enough boy.
At the age of 15 years he seemed to have come to the end
of his tether. Staff at the Assessment Centre before
treatment began perceived him as a boy who was devoid
of any humour, and one who caused them to feel depressed
after a few minutes conversation with him. The one
positive factor in the situation was that the day school he
had been attending was willing to have him back. It
seemed impossible, however, that he could return to his
own home, partly because of the nature and attitude of his
family and the attitude of the local population outside his
home.
A programme was devised which covered, amongst
other things, sex education, social skill training leading
to the ability to go out to youth clubs in the local community, an intensive programme culminating in C.S.E.

examinations, extensive encouragement to join in activities with other boys, and general help in becoming more
independent. In addition, the programme involved intensive casework with the family, including an educative
programme concentrating on the facts of normal maturation at the time of adolescence. After approximately six
months the boy was able to return home and to go back to
his local school. He returned home approximately twelve
months ago. The latest information about him which we
have is that he is doing well, living at home and working
regularly.
Hence the identification of this boy's needs allowed a broad
based, inter-disciplinary service to be provided within the
safety and acceptance of a residential setting.

TEAMWORK

There are many forms of teamwork. We intend to describe
an eclectic approach to residential care using a staff team
made up of representatives from a number of disciplines -
field and residential social work, psychiatry, teaching,
psychology and nursing. It is essential for such a team of
people to maintain a sense of worth and this can be no easy
matter when they are seen by society, or more truthfully,
by vociferous, comparatively small, pressure groups in
society, as failing because the young people are not mirac-
ulously cured of a delinquent way of life when they return
from the residential experience to an unchanged family and
neighbourhood in which the delinquent patterns of behaviour
were originally nurtured. Professional people can perceive success in other areas but in some cases the gains
are small so staff must be able to tolerate the investment of
time, effort and professional skills in return for little
immediate reward. When the children are seriously emotionally or behaviourally disturbed they have typically been
in a number of residential establishments and have been
labelled 'incurable' or 'unhelpable', so in an establishment
catering for these children staff must concentrate on the
positive aspects of their work otherwise they will see themselves as maintaining a 'cordon sanitaire' instead of alleviating serious social and personal handicaps, modifying
anti-social behaviour, and promoting personal growth.
  The residential task should be clarified for this serves
the double purpose of ensuring that the children are given

careful consideration and of demonstrating to the staff
team that professional care, education and treatment can
alleviate the effects of social and personal handicap. The
residential task is seen in different terms for each child
and can be clarified by regular weekly meetings of a task
orientated staff group. Such meetings may be termed case
conferences but what really matters is the value that is
placed upon them, and senior staff have the task of maintaining interest and of demonstrating by their attitudes,
communications and behaviour that the everyday work of the
unit takes into account the individual programmes evolved
from the discussions at case conferences (Gregory, 1980).

   The task orientated group, meeting regularly, helps the
multi-disciplinary team knit together as an effective working unit. Members of the different disciplines must know
that their contributions are valued and the form which the
conference takes is crucial (see Chapter four). When members of different professions meet together for a common
purpose there are bound to be difficulties. Social workers, teachers, nurses, psychologists and psychiatrists
have experienced different forms of training and have qualifications valued at different levels by society. Some
workers are conditioned to feeling that their contributions
are not as valuable as those of more highly paid people.
Underlying conflicts could oppose the group's objectives
unless free and open discussion were possible. Free discussion, through time, reveals that each profession has a
valuable contribution to make and that each can learn from
the other. Well-known conflicts occur again and again but
when they are recognised they are less destructive to the
residential task.

   Residential social workers sometimes reveal a hostile
attitude towards field social workers. Such hostility can
be generated by a number of causal factors such as different salary scales and different professional skills. Residential workers can feel that they are the ones who have
the emotionally draining task of using professional relationships in the residential setting with difficult-to-help, self-
centred, young people for long periods of time and they have
to listen to the pontificating of someone who sees the youngster infrequently for very short periods of time (Dunham,
1978). The field social workers can feel that they are
being misjudged by people who have no idea of the size of
their workload, no idea of the number of hours they work
during evenings and weekends, and certainly no idea of the

importance of involving the family in plans for the child's future. Teachers can be accused by social workers of being too authoritarian in attitude and social workers by teachers of being too permissive and concentrating on the idea of forming easy, superficial relationships with clients (Pritchard and Taylor, 1979). Such feelings can be satis- factorily worked through by a well-functioning, effective staff group.

McGregor (1960) characterises such a group and it is on these lines that attempts have been made to develop the task group. The atmosphere tends to be informal, comfortable and relaxed. There is a lot of discussion in which every member participates but the discussion remains pertinent to the task. The task of the group is well understood and accepted by the members. Members listen to each other and every idea is given a hearing. People do not appear to be afraid of being foolish by putting forward a creative thought even if it seems fairly extreme. There is dis- agreement. Disagreements are not suppressed or over- ridden by premature group action. The reasons are care- fully examined and the group seeks to resolve them rather than to dominate the dissenter. Most decisions are reached by a kind of consensus in which it is clear that everybody is in general agreement. The group does not accept a simple majority as a proper basis for action. Criticism is fre- quent, frank and relatively comfortable. There is little evidence of personal attack, either openly or in a hidden fashion. People are free in expressing their feelings as well as their ideas both on the problem and on the group's operation. When action is taken, clear assignments are made and accepted. The Chairman of the group does not dominate it, nor on the contrary does the group defer un- duly to him. In fact, the leadership shifts from time to time depending on the circumstances. There is little evi- dence of a struggle for power as the group operates. The issue is not who controls but how to get the job done.

A group, taking on these characteristics outlined by McGregor, is well suited to the task of considering the cir- cumstances of a youngster in residential care and evolving an individual programme for his future. The detailed re- cording of the work of this group is essential for communi- cating to staff who are unable to be present, as a reminder of the commitment of staff to various aspects of the child's care, education and treatment, for communicating to inter- ested outside agencies, and for communicating to any future

care establishment or social worker who may become involved.   The staff group then has the responsibility for draw-
ing up a programme designed to be as helpful as possible to
a child and his family, having taken their views into consideration.

THE CONTENT OF RESIDENTIAL CARE

Clare Winnicott makes it quite clear that in her view the
residential worker has a responsibility to provide real experiences of good care, comfort and control: 'These good
experiences are not only the stuff of life, but the stuff that
dreams are made of, and have the power to become part of
the child's inner psychic reality, correcting the past and
creating the future' (Winnicott, 1964, p. 30).   These good
experiences are those which take the place of those normally provided in our society by parents in the family setting.
The experiences are those which are essential to the child's
satisfactory development, those that help the child to learn
the cultural patterns and help the child to grow towards
adulthood, both as an integrated individual and a responsible member of the community.   A residential unit for
adolescent offenders can never take over entirely the work
of parents but it acts as a standby, seeing the youngsters
through emergencies and crises.   In the model of residential care being described acceptance is part of the climate
of the unit which should convey to the adolescents that the
ethos of the establishment is that in each young person admitted there is the possibility of development.   Sound physical care is of prime importance.   Adolescents in residential care should not only receive good food, drink, bodily
comfort and, when necessary, peace, but they should feel
catered for because of the psychological implications of
physical care (Beedell, 1970).
   As has been stated, it is so highly probable that it can
be regarded as certain that there is no way of going about
the residential task that is more important than the people
that are performing the task (Millham, Bullock and Hosie,
1978).   Because of this there must be a consideration of
the use of relationships that develop between adolescents
in residential care and the professional workers engaged
in the task.
   The study described by Ferris (1978) indicates that it is
possible for good professional relationships to have a posi-

tive effect on attitudes, but Hudson (1979) notes the dangers
inherent in pressurising young people into accepting relationships that are not needed by them and in denying necessary relationships to deprived, developing children. If
acceptance is to be part of the climate of a unit then it must
be conveyed in individual relationships. The adolescent
feels accepted when he is valued as an individual by sensitive adults.

The attitudes of the staff as revealed in their day-to-day
behaviour in interaction with each other are also important
where the concept of acceptance is concerned. Hierarchi-
cal staff management which tends to highlight mistakes and
make little of the contributions of individual people does not
help the formation of an accepting climate and has a detri-
mental effect on both staff and children. The relationship
between the adolescent and the residential worker is crucial. This is stated in spite of the fact that many of the
adolescents may be regarded as amoral, unresponsive to
social reinforcement, and as having communication barriers
and a strong determination to reject the adult model presented by the residential worker. The term 'relationship' and
the phrase 'using relationships' are glibly used and because
they mean so many things to different people it can be argued
that they are without any real meaning. Some workers
would vouch for the importance of relationships but would
hesitate to be specific about something which is so personal
and the use of which is so intuitive. For deprived adolescents who have suffered rejection after rejection and have
built up defences to protect themselves from further pain,
but who nevertheless have a basic need for someone to
devote time and attention to them, the concern of a member
of staff becomes one of the most important parts of the total
helping process. According to Adler 'The supreme law (of
life) is this: the sense of worth of the self shall not be
allowed to be diminished.' (Ansbacher and Ansbacher,
1946). For an adolescent whose past experiences have
caused him to view himself as unlovable the need for him to
increase his self-esteem is paramount, and the experience
of his feeling worthy of the long-term care and concern of
an adult is therapeutic.

Without attempting to be exclusive it is possible to say
that a useful professional relationship is formed when the
child's communication with the adult is increased, when the
child becomes more responsive to social reinforcement, and
when the child tends to copy the behaviour of the adult.

Increasing the amount of communication that is not distorted usually means an increase in verbal communication, but
often private words and symbols develop. If the child
begins to want the approval and to avoid the disapproval of
the adult then a way of increasing desired behaviour and
decreasing unwanted behaviour is available. Concrete
reward and punishment is not necessary. This useful professional relationship is not easily achieved and the amount
of influence social approval or disapproval will have upon
behaviour depends mainly on the previous experience of a
child with adults.

Herbert and Jarvis (1961) examined the ways in which it
can be attempted to help delinquent adolescents achieve a
permanent alteration in behaviour by the use of the 'essential relationship'. They stated that a simple definition of
a relationship is that it exists when two people have continuing feelings about each other. These feelings range from
kindly to hostile but the important point is that the worker
must control his feelings and not seek gratification of his
own emotions which should be left to his private life (see
Chapter nine). When the child begins to copy the behaviour
patterns of the adult this is more than seeking approval
since it continues when the adult is not present. This
underlines the responsibility of the worker in residential
establishments for children.

The existence of a relationship places the child in a vulnerable position and he can be influenced for better or for
worse. This can be seen in the case of parents who discipline their child's aggressive behaviour by physically
punishing him and thus provide a model for more physically
aggressive behaviour by the children. The effective residential worker would restrain the aggressive child in a calm
way and through time substitute acceptable behaviour for the
aggressive behaviour. When verbal communication increases it is possible to attempt behavioural modification by insight learning. Total circumstances can be perceived and
discussed and behaviour which causes harm or unhappiness
can be teased out and as a result modified.

However important the professional relationship may be,
if other aspects of residential care are neglected then boredom can result, and in an establishment for adolescents
this is soul destroying. Purposeful outlets for physical
energy are essential and time, space and materials for as
many creative activities as possible should be provided.
An adolescent should have the opportunity, for instance, to

paint, sing, act or play a musical instrument. An adolescent's self-image can be crippling to his development and many adolescents derive status and a sense of achievement in the peer group by delinquent behaviour, and it is of benefit to them to enjoy these pleasurable feelings in acceptable pursuits.

One young man, for instance, was engaged in messing up a group activity which involved reading and when taken to task he blurted out in his own inimitable fashion, 'What do you expect? I can't read.' It is not necessary to have recourse to research which indicates a link between poor reading ability and behavioural difficulties for the sensitive adult to appreciate the predicament of the adolescent who is a poor reader. The residential school for disturbed adolescents needs the teacher who has the special patience, understanding and ability to improve the reading performance of those pupils who have been conditioned to see themselves as unworthy because they failed to learn to read around the time when the vast majority of their contemporaries achieved success in this activity. The poor reader has often entered that vicious circle where he failed to learn to read, was unable to receive the reward of his teacher's approval, failed to learn in other school subjects, earned rejection and ridicule from peers, and became alienated from school and its objectives.

Adolescence is a time for growth providing, as it were, a second chance. The opportunity for making the best use of this growing period should not be wasted. Progress in physical and intellectual development can, in the right circumstances, bring emotional development along in its wake. The inter-disciplinary approach, by its nature, is suited to secure all round development in the adolescent. Teachers teach and use relationships, social workers use relationships and teach, nurses nurse and use relationships, psychiatrists help staff in their professional task and provide treatment where treatment is indicated, and psychologists perform similarly. With teaching techniques that have not failed in the adolescent's past, and individual attention for those who are inhibited by the group, there is no reason why there should not be progress in the basic school subjects for many, and the experience of success for almost all.

It must also be noted that residential care deals with people in groups. A residential institution may therefore, for instance, be asked to deal simultaneously with a with-

drawn, immature neurotic young person and also an aggressive extrovert who has committed extremely serious crimes.
These difficulties are compounded by the fact that the
depths of disturbance and the degree of damage is by no
means necessarily reflected in the presenting behaviour nor
in its management. John and Harold, for example, were
from severely deprived backgrounds and in the same residential unit together. John was excessively tidy, modelling himself on his self-contained father who was the cause
of his own deprivation; he was barely amenable to treatment because of his strong psychological defences. Harold
tested relationships by regressing to infantile behaviour
including soiling, body-rocking, head-banging and thumb
sucking.

A variety of forms of group work can be helpful. The
most immature probably benefit most from group work that
is based on play. Most individuals need to regress occasionally and adolescents who have been deprived of the
usual play possibilities need to regress more than most.
There is no reason why opportunities for such regression
should not be provided. Disruptive adolescents with strong
anti-authority feelings not only need control in group work,
but also the experience of interacting satisfactorily with
adults in positions of authority. Disturbed adolescents who
are able to use words will probably be helped by free discussion groups. If a group of adolescents is too big then
group work becomes counter-productive. The immature
hyperactive youngsters are not able to allow the others to
talk and the most delinquent become the most influential.
A carefully selected group of around six in number can
benefit from the right kind of group work. Role-play, both
planned and spontaneous, can be utilised to help to improve
confidence and competence in social interaction. Improved
verbal ability could result in a reduction in frustration
which had often in the past been relieved by aggressive behaviour. Insight learning can take place by sensitive confrontation, but there should always be respect for the individual's privacy and an awareness of likely behaviour, for
disturbed adolescents in a group have the right to be sure
of adult control.

THE IMPACT ON STAFF

The residential task can be stressful for staff, and there are casualties. However, an inter-disciplinary caring staff team should function in a way that minimises stress and suffering. A staff team is probably strongest if it has a balance of men and women of different ages to provide the widest possible variety of interaction so that the adolescents, by trial and error, can learn appropriate behaviours and become confident in social interaction. Members of staff need to be stable and sure of their sexual roles. Staff must interact with difficult adolescents knowing that they are vulnerable to accusations, particularly of indulging in illegal corporal punishment or illegal or inappropriate sexual behaviour. Experience, if properly used, helps to develop professional practice with in-built awareness and safeguards, but the inexperienced staff member needs help unless he is to learn by the painful experience of suffering accusations and enquiries (Davis, 1977).

The professional relationship does not happen by the light of nature. This is one reason why professional training is so important. It is so easy for the residential worker to lose objectivity, and to find great difficulty in accepting conference recommendations that do not fit in exactly with his own ideas about the treatment of the adolescent with whom he is relating. It has also been known for the trauma of separation to be worse for the staff member than for the adolescent when the time has arrived for parting.

Members of staff have to withstand the testing-out behaviour of adolescents. There are some adolescents whose past experience of lack of certainty of adults' concern has caused them to develop ways of testing this concern which can be hurtful to inexperienced workers. It is sometimes extremely difficult to go along with the notion of accepting the adolescent whilst not condoning the misbehaviour when the misbehaviour is personally hurtful. Staff also have their own personal lives to lead and the personal and domestic relationships which matter to them can be affected if the difficult relationships at work take up too much energy. If the professional worker fails to balance his contribution he is liable to suffer from stress and become less effective (Dunham, 1978).

When working with children in trouble staff have to keep the children in touch with reality, with their families, and

with happenings in their neighbourhoods. There are times
when staff find it difficult to accept decisions which they do
not consider helpful to the adolescent because of demands
from individuals, agencies or other sources in the community.

The inter-disciplinary approach that has been briefly
described hopefully helps the adolescents and minimises
stress in staff, but it is an expensive form of residential
care which should be reserved for particularly disturbed
and damaged adolescents, for, as West states: 'Institutions
are too often run to suit the least disturbed, who are capable of responding favourably to ordinary methods, whereas
of course it is the worst cases who should get the best
attention' (West, 1967, p. 297).

CONCLUSION

We have attempted to examine some of the ways in which
social work can be deployed in residential settings. Attention has been drawn to the many conflicting factors which
can be present at the same time. It has also been pointed
out that residential social work has to be concerned with a
number of individuals within a group setting. Because of
the differing needs of the individuals, skills are necessary
at varying levels. We have described some practical
approaches to residential social work. We have demonstrated how it is possible to break up the overall task into
manageable short term goals and to closely monitor results.
It is also possible to assess and work at the complex task
in its entirety by using the child-centred approach of an
interactive multi-disciplinary staff team.

Finally, we would like to draw attention to the enormous
stresses on staff doing residential social work with adolescents, and some of these issues are explored further in the
next chapter. However, the work can be the most fruitful
and rewarding of all, but only to those social workers pos-
sessing the necessary basic human qualities.

Chapter nine

Some common problems in working with adolescents

Kenneth E. Reid

/This paper explores, from a predominantly psychodynamic
perspective and based upon experience of social work in the
USA, some of the issues and difficulties which may personally confront the social worker in face-to-face work with
adolescents. Although the discussion focuses on the adolescent and the counsellor, we feel it is relevant to all those
adults, including social workers, who are involved with
young people. The chapter examines how the social worker
may attempt to satisfy some of his own needs through his
interaction with the adolescent. It also describes some of
the personal traumas which may face the social worker who
is directly involved with young people. The paper concludes with some thoughts on those aspects of worker style
which may lead to effective counselling./

It has long been recognised that adolescents, as a whole,
are a group that social workers and psychotherapists alike
approach with trepidation and reluctance, or avoid altogether. There are several reasons for this unwillingness.
In the first place, counsellors, while trained to deal mainly
with children and adults, are not particularly well equipped
to work with young people between the ages of 12 and 18.
When workers use techniques that are normally effective
with children, they find themselves talking down to the adolescents and if the worker utilises methods used with adults,
they seem to go over the adolescent's head.
  Likewise, the adolescent's attitude toward counselling
differs from that of younger and older clients. A child referred for help will often perceive the worker as a trusted
playmate, and enjoy the attention he receives. Adult
clients, if they want counselling, are ready to work in the

counselling sessions, even though they may have ambivalent feelings. The adolescent, on the other hand, may have been dragged to the agency by a well-meaning parent. They may not admit to having problems and do not want to be there. Their initial attitude is often that of 'treat me, I dare you!'

Another reason professionals resist working with adolescents has to do with the fact that the youngster's behaviour often becomes a threat to the worker's own emotional economy. The challenging, competitive, depreciating, provocative, and volatile adolescent can elicit anxiety, defensiveness, and doubt in adults who are generally self-assured. Many youngsters are extremely adept at ferreting out the hidden emotional vulnerability and blind spots all workers have. For these and other reasons, counselling adolescents has the potential for being the most 'challenging, the most frustrating and the most baffling experience a worker can have' (Josselyn, 1952, p. 76).

The focus of this chapter is on this third issue, the impact of the adolescent on the counsellor and the counselling process. Unless the worker is aware of the dynamics of the client-worker interaction, there is a real likelihood of failure. By contrast, if the worker is attuned to the dynamics that are present within the helping relationship and aware of his own needs, he is in a much better position to manage the situation effectively and therapeutically.

FORMING THE THERAPEUTIC ALLIANCE

An issue with which the social worker is confronted in the early stages of the treatment process is that of determining the extent of the adolescent's difficulties. While it is unlikely that the worker will be in a position of having to establish a specific clinical diagnosis, as might a psychologist or a psychiatrist, he will be required to discriminate between those behaviours that are transient and linked to the youngster's particular stage of development, and those which are more long term in nature and possibly require hospitalisation. Fritz Redl has summed up the situation thus:

> One of the problems those of us face who are supposed to be helpful to adolescents by means of 'counselling' or 'therapy' was clearly recognized by Anna Freud, and has baffled us ever since. If I may state it somewhat crudely

and as briefly as possible: How do I know whether whatever they do is simply 'because they are going through a
developmental phase' or whether they are on the verge of
going crazy, or of becoming juvenile delinquents? Or
worse even, maybe the problem behaviour producer this
morning falls into the 'crazy' category while similar behaviour by the same kid in the afternoon belongs to the
'hard to live with but basically normal' category? (Redl,
1975, p. xv).

For some adolescents referred to social agencies have always displayed evidence of disturbed behaviour, and possibly would have arrived much sooner had it not been for
the fact that their actions had been assumed to be something
that would diminish if ignored, or something they would just
'outgrow'. Other youngsters, struggling reasonably well
with their lives, begin to show problems as a response to
external traumatic events. Still, the majority of the adolescents seen in counselling are suffering from specific
adolescent stresses. Their problems are precipitated by
the onset of adolescence and the tasks inherent in that
period. Their conflicts are not purely adolescent but
rather activate and highlight points of relative weakness in
the personality structure.

In the past clinicians have been quick to label adolescents as sociopathic or schizophrenic without anticipating
the actual meaning this categorisation may have for the individual. Increasingly, however, it is coming to be recognised that because of the adolescent's susceptibility to the
expectations of others, labels of this nature tend to be
damning rather than useful. Since the troubled adolescent
may be unsure as to what he is, he may identify with, and
become, someone whose problems are chronic and whose
prognosis is poor. For this reason, workers in both
Great Britain and the USA are becoming increasingly cautious in the use of labels and in their attitude towards
youngsters' problems (see Menninger, 1963).

Another problem in developing a working alliance with an
adolescent client is that of dealing with the negativism which
seems to be so common to adolescents. It would be nice to
think that when the client meets the worker he will be open,
interested and willing to share his concerns and conflicts.
Unfortunately, this is usually not the case. Adolescents
are often particularly fearful of the therapeutic situation
and its ambiguity. A somewhat anxious 17-year-old girl,
commenting on her personal feelings in an interview, remar-

ked, 'Once the door is closed, I feel I am on stage and there is no place to hide.'

Each youngster will deal with the lack of predictability and the ambiguity of the situation differently, based on a combination of factors including their previous experience with adults, especially those in authority, and cultural and subgroup norms. If the youngster has, through past experience, found adults to be undependable and manipulative, it can be anticipated that he will expect the same thing of the worker. Likewise, if this basic distrust is reinforced regularly by his peer group who are having similar experiences, it is inevitable that the worker, no matter how well skilled or well meaning, will be confronted with negativsim, suspicion and anxiety.

Some youngsters defend themselves against the anxiety of the situation by remaining silent, thereby putting the responsibility of the interview on the shoulders of the worker. All seasoned social workers have, at some point in their career, had the painful experience of sitting across from a youngster who has chosen to be verbally noncommunicative. The worker's statements and questions are responded to in the same manner - either silence or monosyllables. After ten minutes to the monologue, the worker feels angry and after fifteen minutes he begins to feel inadequate. If by some unfortunate coincidence he should run into the same kind of response on the same day with another youngster, the professional may begin to question whether or not he is cut out to work with anyone under 21.

Because referrals are usually made by adults through agency channels, it is natural for the youngster to feel little or no control of his life. He senses collusion and conspiracy, with him being the victim. Silence, therefore, becomes a very powerful weapon to keep his 'attackers' away. By not sharing his thoughts verbally he has control over this potentially dangerous and threatening situation.

If the adolescent comes to the attention of the agency through a referral from the court, schools or other state institution, the worker feels caught between two powerful forces. The community wants him to control or in some way modify the behaviour of the youth who is causing it some distress. The worker is also interested in his client and wants to assist him to achieve a higher and more meaningful level of functioning. The community pays the worker's salary and when the community's needs come into conflict with the adolescent's, it is the youngster who usually loses.

PROFESSIONAL DISHONESTY

Workers in the helping professions consider themselves
honest, reliable and trustworthy. Few would admit to
lying, manipulating or deceiving their clients. However,
when one looks closely at the transactions that occur in
adolescent counselling, it becomes apparent that a significant amount of dishonesty takes place. Halleck (1963), in
calling attention to this issue, writes that adolescent clients
are deceived either through conscious fabrications or
through subtle and unconscious communication of attitudes
to which professional workers do not adhere. The net
effect of this behaviour, according to Halleck, is to confuse and at times to infuriate the adolescent which, in
itself, may produce greater rebellion, more symptoms, and
increased pain.

One such form of professional dishonesty is the 'lie of
adult morality' in which adult counsellors communicate a
picture of themselves and their world as one in which only
the highest types of values and moral standards prevail.
This is contrary to the adolescent's personal experience,
his observational powers, and intuitiveness which tells him
that something is wrong. He wants to like and identify with
adults but he is painfully aware of the inconsistency and
basic dishonesty in their approach. He may then come to
believe that adults are incapable of being anything but
phoney and react by rebellion or isolation from the adult
world.

Another form of professional dishonesty is the myth,
'open up; trust me; and all will go well.' For many youngsters, lowering their defences and putting their trust in an
adult is mixed with danger, threat, and risk. He knows
that the person who is pleading with him to expose himself
may be someone with whom he will have only limited future
contact and whom he can see few reasons for trusting. He
is further aware of the possibility that he can lose much in
such a relationship and the worker may not be offering a
true intimacy between equals. To the adolescent, this may
seem like a poor bargain. He feels the worker is dishonest
in affecting this type of bargain and he reacts with fear,
mistrust, and cynicism.

The majority of adolescents who are in contact with social
workers and counsellors come from lower socio-economic
groups. Many are from broken homes and have been subjected to painful psychological and economic deprivations.

Their parents may have received little schooling and their own educational experience may also have been limited. Because of early emotional deprivation, certain aspects of their intellectual capacity may be restricted and unmodifiable (see Bowlby, 1958; Harlow, 1958).

The average professional worker, in contrast, comes from a white, middle-class background which tends to provide greater opportunities and encouragement for advancement than that which the adolescent has experienced. Workers fail to see that often they are dealing with individuals who may never be able to achieve the same level of life they have (Halleck, 1963). Failing to realise this, they may then encourage identifications, ambitions and achievements that are not possible for the client and which leave the adolescent feeling frustrated and inadequate.

ADOLESCENT'S IMPACT ON THE WORKER

It is naïve to think that the counsellor has influence on the adolescent's life without recognising that the adolescent also has impact on the worker's life. Their dress, attitudes, and values all have the power of triggering non-rational feelings and actions on the worker's part. Never static, this reaction will not only vary from client to client but from session to session. To some clients the worker may demonstrate feelings of affection, while to others he may find himself feeling bored, irritated, and even hostile. Such responses are more or less automatic, being nurtured by motives that operate outside the awareness of the worker (see Reid, 1977).

Attack on traditional values

The adolescent's volatility, narcissism, lack of commitment, irreverence, and acting out behaviour may be as discomforting to the worker as it is for the parents. It is no mistake that youngsters seem to question and attack those values that adults tend to consider important such as those derived from religion, tradition, status and the vague, coercive strength of the 'establishment'. The worker unaware of his own sensitivity may find the adolescent's challenge of traditional values disturbing, and his sense of discomfort and outrage may block any effort to treat the adolescent.

The counsellor who is still actively struggling with his
own identity and is still in rebellion against cultural values
may be no better prepared to deal with the adolescent. He
may inflame the youngster's natural tendency toward icono-
clasm and overlook the more important 'civil-war' within the
client, which can only be resolved successfully through
compromise and accommodation to psychological reality.
The uncertain worker, according to Meeks (1971), may go
even further, abdicating his responsibility and looking to
the adolescent to provide him with a workable ideology in a
changing cultural scene. This unfortunate reversal can
only result in chaos, not just in the therapeutic situation,
but in the adolescent.

Worker's past experiences

One thing the worker has in common with the adolescent
client is the fact that he, too, has gone through adolescence.
This period in the worker's life may have been relatively
uneventful in the sense that there were few serious crises
and a minimum amount of stress, or adolescence may have
been painful with some aspects still left unresolved.   In
the latter case, the client's reports of his own experience
may resurrect significant issues that had been forgotten
or buried at an unconscious or preconscious level.
An example of this is the adolescent of the same sex who
becomes the vehicle for the accomplishment of frustrated
self-expression.   Where the worker has been unable to
reach his own personal goal, the client, benefited by the
worker's sage advice and counsel, may succeed. Equally
disruptive is the situation where the worker feels defensive
regarding his own deficiencies.   The adolescent client becomes a threat, with the worker fearful the younger person
will surpass him.
The social worker, whether working with children, adolescents, or adults, needs to be content with his own life,
age level, and past experiences. This includes a comfortable awareness of the areas of his life in which he is disappointed with himself. Achieving personal maturity always
includes facing up to the many ambitions that have not been
realised and mourning some fantasies which have never been
gratified in reality.

LIVING VICARIOUSLY THROUGH THE CLIENT

One of the most dangerous temptations for the worker is
that of using the adolescent to gratify their own libidinal
needs. Although it is probably extremely rare for a
worker to actually act out their sexual feelings toward the
client, it is not unusual for them to participate vicariously
in their sexual behaviour. Evidence of this type of living
through the client appears in the form of humour, fantasies,
and therapeutic blunders.

The client and the worker are at different stages in their
personal development. For the adolescent, this is a time
of sexual discovery and experimentation. They are becoming increasingly aware of their own feelings and are struggling with their sexual role. Interlaced with these feelings of discovery may be the feelings of anxiety about their
personal adequacy and their ability to maintain a meaningful
relationship with members of the opposite sex.

The social workers, on the other hand, passed the discovery and experimentation stage several years earlier
and have progressed to the building and consolidation stage.
They are established as professionals and feel increased
stability and confidence in their role as social workers.
Physically, they are beginning to recognise that they no
longer have the same stamina and endurance they had ten
years earlier. Their own children may be entering adolescence and gradually moving from being completely dependent to becoming independent. Their sexual relationship
with their spouse may be satisfactory but no longer filled
with the same excitement and spontaneity that was once
present (see Sheehy, 1977).

It is certainly not surprising that the adolescent is capable of stirring suppressed yearnings in the worker. Not
only is the healthy and vigorous youngster attractive as a
sexual object, but seems to be living a life of freedom and
sensuality that is most appealing. When this mythical image
is linked to the adult's nostalgic mourning for missed opportunities, there is the potential for real danger.

A 40-year-old colleague spoke of his discomfort with a
female adolescent client in the following way:
'It is really frustrating to sit here week after week listening to her talk about her relationship with her boy-
friend. I really envy them. While they worry whether
or not to go to a disco, or bike trip, the big thing in my
life is deciding on what colour to paint the bedroom.

Sometimes I think I should get the hell out of here, grow
a beard and live off the land. I've got a good wife, nice
kids, and an expensive house, but I'm bored.'
What is needed is not total freedom from such disquieting
feelings, but rather a comfortable awareness that they are
present, natural and, more importantly, that they are illu-
sory. If the worker does not have a clear picture of what
is going on inside the helping relationship, he can easily
lose his professional perspective.

THE LOSS OF INVOLVED IMPARTIALITY

Through training and experience the worker learns the important lesson that they must remain emotionally controlled
when working with clients. They are to become involved in
the client's life but at the same time keep their distance so
as not to over-identify or side with one person against another. When working with an adolescent in individual counselling, it is easy to lose this impartiality, especially when
it is impossible to view the adolescent's relationships and
roles in other situations.
The most common example of this is the worker siding
with the client who appears to be victimised by other members of the family. This author attended a workshop in
which a well-known psychiatrist demonstrated his particular brand of therapy to an audience of social workers. As
part of the programme he interviewed a young man who
appeared quite despondent. During an hour-long interview,
the client hesitantly told how he was harassed by his family
and not allowed the same rights and privileges as the other
members. The more he spoke the more the therapist (and
the audience) identified with the young man's struggle. It
was decided, with great moral indignation, that the parents
should also be interviewed. When they arrived, there was
some surprise by everyone in attendance that neither the
mother nor the father had cloven hoofs or a tail. As they
told their side of the story it became apparent that the therapist (and the audience) had been taken in to the point of
forgetting there may have been another viewpoint. The
young man had been able to 'hook' into the group's 'rescue
fantasies' so that it was no longer his struggle but theirs.
There was complete loss of objectivity with the professional
completely identified with the victim.
Rebellious adolescents who are constantly in conflict with

adults pose similar problems for the worker.   Rather than
the worker protecting the client from the family and significant others as previously described, the worker becomes
the spokesman for the rebellion.   He is constantly in the
role of explaining what the behaviour means and becomes the
middleman between the youngster and his parents.

The motivational dynamics of the worker vary.   Stierling,
in discussing one form of siding in young therapists, writes
the following:

> Through their dress, e.g. slightly frayed jeans and
> manner of hippie talk, they document visibly their identi-
> fication with the protesting young generation.   Having not
> yet achieved a more mature dependence (or independence
> if you wish) in relation to their own parents, they recruit
> their patients to unwittingly and vicariously continue their
> own 'rebellious' struggle (Stierling, 1975, p. 161).

Siding with the victim is not limited to the worker identifying with the adolescent (see Chapter five).   Workers often
side with the parent against the youngster.   Here the siding
worker over identifies with the much maligned, misunderstood parent against the 'spoiled' obstreperous adolescent.
It is not uncommon under these circumstances for the worker
to encourage the victimised parents to drastic punishment
under the rubric of firmness and limit setting.   Rather than
assisting the parents to stand firm, he only supports the rejecting, hostile side in their, and his own, ambivalence,
thereby courting disaster.   The more the parents reject
and punish, the more they also alienate their youngster; the
very thing they are trying to overcome.

PREREQUISITES TO EFFECTIVE COUNSELLING

The client often comes to the counselling situation in a
state of alienation from his parents and from the internalised sanctions and ideals which have been derived from them.
He needs a trusted friend outside the family situation who
will listen without being judgmental or controlling.   Unfortunately in a society characterised by isolation, overcrowd-
ing, impersonal classrooms, and neighbourhoods with de-
clining social cohesion, there may be few opportunities to
develop such a relationship.

It should be no surprise that a majority of youngsters
long for an adult who will listen and answer troubling questions that haunt them.   Adolescents still worry that they

may be sexually abnormal despite the increase in sexual sophistication. They are fearful of their sexual impulses, size and appearance of genitals, personal attractiveness, and body size and shape (see Chapter two). These questions can rarely be settled by education alone since they are often rooted in unconscious conflicts. Truthful answers from someone they trust at least helps the adolescent to distinguish those concerns which are realistic from those that are related to personal problems.

For effective change to occur, the worker must learn to conduct the counselling sessions in a reasonably relaxed conversational style. Few adolescents can tolerate a silent, totally passive 'blank screen' technique or a stiff and stilted style of counselling. The reaction to the worker's silence and formality is usually that of anxiety and increased defensiveness. The practical dilemma for the worker becomes that of being reasonably talkative and responsive without being directive or intrusive. It is also important that the worker avoid comments and remarks that the adolescent has heard from parents or adults with whom he is having difficulty.

The single most important tool available for working with young adults is the worker himself, sensitive, trained and dedicated to the helping tasks. In each encounter with the adolescent the worker has to present a self capable of being many things to a multi-faceted and changing client, who needs someone he can rely and depend upon during his struggle between dependence and independence. The worker may be one of the few adults with whom the adolescent has come into contact who is stable, consistent, and predictable.

The worker must be capable of entering the helping relationship without anything of himself to prove or protect. He needs to convey to the client an openness, and realness, and unconditional positive regard. He needs to be able to relate to the client without front or façade, openly expressing the feelings and attitudes that are flowing inside him.

This means that at certain times the worker may be very direct with the client telling him exactly what he is feeling. For example, if the worker is experiencing anger, it may be appropriate to share it with the adolescent. It is surprisingly easy to tell a youngster when he is annoying and such communications, when presented in a non-hostile manner, rarely have a negative effect on the relationship. A statement such as 'I find your behaviour extremely difficult, and it is beginning to bother me' is often more useful than questions such as 'What's bothering you?' or 'How can I help you?'

Finally, it is important for the worker to be scrupulously honest with the adolescent. By the time the worker comes to his first meeting with the youngster, he is encountering an individual who has probably been lied to frequently by his parents, relatives, and also, possibly, by other workers, such as teachers, the police, and other social workers.

From his experience, the child may have learned a variety of techniques of resistance to cope with what he perceives to be the 'phoniness' and manipulation of the adult world. This may be one of the most important causes of sullen inertia, negativism, and defiance which are so much a part of the adolescent life style. Many of the malignant effects of this factor can be diminished through a change in techniques and attitudes on the part of the worker. When there is a sincere effort to be honest with adolescent clients, it is likely that the response will be a more open communicative youngster.

A CONCLUDING THOUGHT

The social worker counselling adolescent clients must be comfortable enough with himself to leave aside any pomposity or excessive professional dignity. The youngster will quickly and accurately recognise these as evidence of personal insecurity on the worker's part. As such, they will frighten the adolescent, since his own self-esteem is unsure and he is looking to the worker for strength, dependability and acceptance. These attributes are most effectively conveyed by a simple, honest presentation of oneself as an ordinary person who is also in the process of growing and developing as an individual. This does not mean that the worker denies his training or rational status as an expert, but rather that he avoids claiming any special consideration or adulation as a human being.

Chapter ten

Postscript

Ray Jones and Colin Pritchard

This book has examined a number of practical and theoretical issues concerned with social work for adolescents.
This, in turn, has explicitly posed questions, such as
which theories and what 'methods' might be used, and, im-
plicitly, what is the rationale for a social work service for
adolescents? Let us briefly explore this latter question,
and the associated corollaries for research and training.

THE TASK OF SOCIAL WORK WITH ADOLESCENTS

The task for social work is still one for debate and refine-
ment (CCETSW, 1975; BASW, 1976), though the themes of
comfort, change and control are established as parts of the
social work task. The special task for social work with
adolescents, in addition to those above, is also to be concerned with prevention. By this we mean there is need for
a social work service that not only aims to bring comfort in
a distressing situation; change within an individual or his
social environment; control to a self-destructive crisis or
of intolerable behaviour; but also to seek to prevent a deterioration that may lead to a young person becoming a victim of 'labelling' by an inadequate service, or ultimately
becoming a part of the sad catalogue of psycho-social problems in adulthood.
    It might be argued that stressing the preventative role in
contemporary social work agencies, especially in statutory
agencies, is unrealistic in the current crisis of resources.
Yet we believe that the case for preventative work is overwhelming, despite the disappointments about such programmes; the evidence that a large number of adult psycho-

social casualties also had a problematic childhood and adolescence is extensive. The formidable list includes: child
abuse (Spinetta and Rigler, 1972; Blumberg, 1974); suicide and attempted suicide (McCullough and Philip, 1972;
Kreitman, 1977); behaviour described as psychopathic
(Hare and Schalling, 1978); prison inmate populations
(Stratta, 1970; Prins, 1973); and delinquents who continue
their ciminality into adulthood (West and Farrington, 1977).
  These findings suggest to us the necessity for social work
to recognise the importance of a preventative focus. We
are, however, aware of the difficulties which arise from
this statement (see Rutter, 1978). First, it is not suggested that all adolescents in difficulty subsequently find themselves as a part of adult morbidity statistics; nor are we
assuming that we can predict all of those adolescents who
will continue to experience or create more acute or chronic
difficulties in adulthood. We are also aware that token preventative work can increase the stigma of an adolescent in
difficulties, and that this can promote continued difficulties
in later life. In order to overcome such problems it is
essential, therefore, that social work monitors and eval-
uates its effectiveness; that it incorporates into its practice those elements of intervention which are found to be
effective and helpful; and that it discards those techniques
and approaches which are found to be negative in their
impact on clients. That social work can be effective in
helping young people is suggested by research on detached
youth work (Smith et al., 1972), school counselling (Rose
and Marshall, 1974), and by the differential impact on young
people of varying school regimes (Rutter et al., 1979).
There is, however, also a mass of research which highlights the ineffectiveness, and sometimes the negative
effects, of some types of social work practice (see, for
instance, in the field of delinquency control, Lerman, 1975,
and Lipton et al., 1975).
  So what aspects of social work practice seem to have a
positive impact on clients? Fischer (1978), in a wide-
ranging review of research on the 'helping professions',
noted two areas of practice where an array of positive
findings have accrued. First, he notes that practice based
on the principles of behaviour modification has frequently
led to success in changing certain behaviours (see Lazarus,
1974, and Chapter five). Possibly we could associate with
these findings the positive results from research on task-
centred work (Reid and Shyne, 1969; Reid and Epstein,

1977).   Second, Fischer noted that there is now a good
deal of research which supports the importance for effectiveness of warmth, empathy, and genuineness in the helping process (see, for example, Truax and Carkuff, 1967).
Conversely there is evidence that practitioner pessimism
can be a major stumbling block to effective social work
(Smale, 1977).   In addition it should be noted that indirect
work on behalf of a client, or a group of clients, may sometimes be more effective than direct face-to-face work.   For
example, Thorpe and his colleagues (1979) look at ways in
which the juvenile justice system might be better managed
as a primary way of helping young offenders, whose delinquency is often transitory and petty.

The task, therefore, for the social work practitioner is
to incorporate into his practice those elements of intervention which are shown to be useful; the task for the social
work educator is to train practitioners to use these more
positive techniques and approaches; and the task for the
researcher is to develop methods to monitor and evaluate
practice, and therefore aid in the identification of what is
most efficacious.   These are by no means easy tasks!
But they are tasks which cannot be discarded because there
are methodological problems in researching intervention,
or because in many agencies organisational expediency may
overrule practice efficiency and effectiveness.

There are, however, three points that we would stress.
First, social work must be kept in perspective.   What can
be demanded of social work and social workers must be
limited.   In the lives of our clients, and in the communities
in which they live, we are likely to be a very minor influence compared to other variables, such as the quality of
housing and education, or the provision of health and income
maintenance services.   There are, for instance, only about
28,000 field and residential social workers in jobs which
demand direct contact with clients in England and Wales,
far fewer than, for example, either doctors or nurses
(Merrison Report, 1979).

Second, if the expectations of social work continue to be
confused, perhaps reflecting the conflict and tension within
current social values, it will be impossible to convince all
the sceptics of the usefulness of social work.

Third, while it seems to us that social work can be
effective, the predicament of social work is similar to that
described by Mittler (1971) in regard to environmental factors and the causation of mental illness.   It is difficult to

isolate, measure, and control for all those factors, although they undoubtedly exist. This is also the dilemma
in evaluating those practice components which lead to
successful social work.

EVALUATING RESEARCH

Having stressed the likely need for social workers to
modify their practice to take account of evidence on the differential effectiveness of the various elements included in
social work intervention, it is also necessary for social
workers to be able to evaluate the validity and reliability
of any research. The importance of examining research
critically is exemplified by a seminal study by Eysenck
(1952), which had a cumulative and demoralising impact on
those in the 'helping professions'. Eysenck examined the
therapeutic results of three eminent Freudian psychotherapists, and he found little to recommend their form of treatment. The findings of this research have been unquestion-
ingly accepted by many subsequent writers (for example
Segal, 1972, and Fischer, 1978), who also found little
encouragement from Eysenck's research for social work
intervention. However, when Dührssen and Jorswieck
(1962) re-examined Eysenck's work, by going back to the
original studies, they found serious discrepancies in his
data and his argument. This led them to conclude that
Eysenck had profoundly misinterpreted his statistics. When
replying to the criticism of his research Eysenck failed, in
our view, to deal satisfactorily with the substantive criticisms made (Eysenck, 1964).
    There are two points to be drawn from this example.
First, research should be read critically, and the methodology and data, as well as the researcher's conclusions,
need to be examined. Second, analysis of practice needs
to be able to identify which techniques within a practice
approach are effective or ineffective, rather than just seeking global judgments of success or failure. Only in this
way can practice be refined and improved.

PRACTICE AND POLICY

Finally we would want to comment on the relationship between practice and policy. By practice we mean what the

social worker does; by policy we mean here those wider influences on our clients which also affect their lives. We
have already stated that the contribution that social work
can make to the well-being of individuals and communities
is bound to be limited, as there are wider social factors
which have a major impact on our clients. We feel it is a
responsibility of social workers to comment on these issues.
    We will briefly consider just one problem which especially
concerns us at the present time.· This is the prevalence of
unemployment, especially amongst older adolescents, which
creates particular difficulties for young people. These
difficulties are not only financial, but are also likely to be
social and emotional. We are concerned, for example, at
the conflict which may occur in some families as parents
criticise their children for being out of work. Far from
the intergenerational promise of familial social mobility
which was offered by the boom years of the late 1950s and
the early 1960s, families are now having to face the stigma
and stress of what may be perceived as downward social
mobility, due to unemployment, between the parents' and the
adolescents' generations (Jahoda, 1979). The temporary
relief programmes of the Manpower Services Commission,
while valuable in the short term, offer no solution to continuing structural unemployment. The solutions to this
social problem, as with so many of the difficulties experienced by our clients, are more likely to depend on changes
in social values (for example, the work ethic), and in social
policy (moving towards limited employment for all, rather
than full employment for some and no employment for others).
The solutions to unemployment are economic and political,
and although this book cannot focus on these more general
structural problems, we end, as we began, by stating their
importance. It is these issues which largely determine the
task of practitioners, and which highlight the limited goals
which can be set for social work. But, as we feel this
book has illustrated, although the goals for social work may
be limited, they are certainly not unworthy.

Bibliography

ABRAMS, M. (1959) 'The Teenage Consumer', London
Press Exchange.
ACKERMAN, N.W. (1958) 'The Psychodynamics of Family
Life', Basic Books.
ADELSON, J., GREEN, B. and O'NEIL, R. (1969) Growth
of the Idea of Law in Adolescence, 'Developmental Psychol-
ogy', 1.4, pp. 327-32.
ADELSON, J. and O'NEIL, R. (1966) Growth of Political
Ideas in Adolescence, 'Journal of Personality and Social
Psychology', 4.3, pp. 295-306.
ADVISORY COUNCIL ON THE TREATMENT OF OFFEN-
DERS (1962) 'Non-Residential Treatment of Offenders
under 21', HMSO.
ALLEN, D. (1977) The Residential Task - Is There One?,
'Social Work Today', 9.7, pp. 20-1.
ANDRY, R. (1960) 'Delinquency and Parental Pathology',
Methuen.
ANON. (1975) A Boring Old Talk, 'Youth Social Work Bul-
letin', 2.3, pp. 10-13.
ANSBACHER, H. and ANSBACHER, R. (1946) 'The Indi-
vidual Psychology of Alfred Adler', Harper & Row.
APLIN, G. and BAMBER, R. (1973) Groupwork Counsel-
ling, 'Social Work Today', 3.22, pp. 6-10.
APPLEY, M.H. and TRUMBULL, R. (1967) 'Psychological
Stress', Appleton-Century-Crofts.
ARMSTRONG, G. and WILSON, M. (1973a) City Politics
and Deviancy Amplification, in I. Taylor and L. Taylor
(eds), 'Politics and Deviance', Penguin.
ARMSTRONG, G. and WILSON, M. (1973b) Delinquency and
Some Aspects of Housing, in C. Ward (ed.), 'Vandalism',
Architectural Press.

ATTLEE, C. (1920) 'The Social Worker', Bell.
BAKER, R. (1976) 'The Interpersonal Process in Generic
Social Work: An Introduction', Preston Institute of Tech-
nology, Australia.
BALDOCK, P. (1974) 'Community Work and Social Work',
Routledge & Kegan Paul.
BALDWIN, J. (1977) Why Groupwork?, 'Social Work Today',
8.19, pp. 6-8.
BANDURA, A. (1967) The Role of Modelling Processes in
Personality Development, in J.M. Foley, B. Byrne and D.
Nelson (eds), 'Contemporary Readings in Psychology',
Harper & Row.
BANDURA, A. (1970) The Stormy Decade: Fact or Fic-
tion, in R. Grinder (ed.), 'Studies in Adolescence', Mac-
millan.
BART, P. (1969) Why Women's Status Changes in Middle
Age: The Turns of the Social Ferris Wheel, 'Sociological
Symposium', 3, pp. 1-18.
BART, P. (1971) Depression in Middle-Aged Women, in V.
Gornick and B.K. Morans (eds), 'Women in Sexist Society',
Basic Books.
BASW (1976) 'The Social Work Task', BASW.
BASW (1977) 'The Children and Young Persons Act 1969:
Some Implications for Practice', BASW.
BEEDELL, C. (1970) 'Residential Life with Children',
Routledge & Kegan Paul.
BELSON, W. (1978) 'Television Violence and the Adoles-
cent Boy', Saxon House.
BENSON, J. (1976) The Concept of Community, in N.
Timms and J. Watson (eds), 'Talking About Welfare', Rout-
ledge & Kegan Paul.
BERG, I., NICHOLS, K. and PRITCHARD, C. (1969)
School Phobia - Its Classification and Relationship to
Dependency, 'Journal of Child Psychology and Psychiatry',
10, pp. 123-41.
BERGER, P.L. and LUCKMANN, T. (1972) 'The Social
Construction of Reality', Penguin.
BLAND, G.A. (1976) personal communication.
BLEASDALE, A. (1975) 'Scully', Hutchinson.
BLEULER, M. (1974) The Off-Spring of Schizophrenics,
'Schizophrenia Bulletin', 8, pp. 93-108.
BLOS, P. (1962) 'On Adolescence', Free Press.
BLUMBERG, M.L. (1974) Psychopathology of the Abusing
Parent, 'American Journal of Psychotherapy', 18, pp. 21-9.
BOTTOMS, A.E. (1976) Crime in a City, 'New Society',
8 April, pp. 64-6.

BOWERMAN, C.E. and KINCH, J.W. (1959) Changes in Family and Peer Orientation of Children between the Fourth and Tenth Grades, 'Social Forces', 37, pp. 206-11.

BOWLBY, J. (1958) A Note on Mother-Child Separation as a Mental Health Hazard, 'British Journal of Medical Psychology', 31.3, pp. 3-4.

BRANDON, D. (1976) 'Zen in the Art of Helping', Routledge & Kegan Paul.

BRENNAN, T., HUIZINGA, D. and ELLIOT, D.S. (1978) 'The Social Psychology of Runaways', Lexington.

BREWER, C. (1975) Technical Trappings, 'New Psychiatry', 2.66, pp. 14-15.

BRUNEL UNIVERSITY (1976) Collaboration between Health and Social Services, 'Working Paper, Institute of Organisation and Social Studies', November.

BRYERS, P. (1979) The Development of Practice Theory in Community Work, outline of a paper presented to a 'Workshop on Making Sense of Community Work', organised by Association of Community Workers and National Institute for Social Work, Bristol, March.

BURCK, C. (1978) A Study of Family Expectations and Experiences of a Child Guidance Clinic, 'British Journal of Social Work', 8.2, pp. 145-58.

BURLAND, R. and MATHER, M. (1978) Teaching Alternative Behaviours, 'Therapeutic Education', 6.12, pp. 21-5.

BURNS, J.L. (1977) The Expectations of Residential Care and Alternatives, 'The Community Home Schools Gazette', 70.10, pp. 451-62.

BUTRYM, Z. (1976) 'The Nature of Social Work', Macmillan.

BUTTON, L. (1974) 'Developmental Groupwork with Adolescents', Hodder & Stoughton.

BYNG-HALL, L. and BRUGGEN, P. (1974) Family Admission Decisions as a Therapeutic Tool, 'Family Process', 13.4, pp. 21-30.

CCETSW (1975) 'Education and Training for Social Work', Paper 10, CCETSW.

CCETSW (1978) 'Good Enough Parenting', CCETSW.

CERNY, L. (1977) Ten Years of the Telephone Emergency Service for Children and Youth (Prague), 'Acta Paedopsychiatrica', 42.6, pp. 214-23.

CHEETHAM, J. (1977) 'Unwanted Pregnancy and Counselling', Routledge & Kegan Paul.

CLARE, A. (1976) 'Psychiatry in Dissent: Controversial Issues in Thought and Practice', Tavistock.

CLARK, R.M. (1968) Group Simulation Games and Role
Play, in R.M. Clark (ed.), 'Strategies and Tactics in
Secondary School', Macmillan.
CLARKE, J. (1976) Style, in S. Hall and T. Jefferson
(eds), 'Resistance Through Rituals', Hutchinson.
CLARKE, J. and JEFFERSON, T. (1976) Working Class
Youth Cultures, in G. Mungham and G. Pearson (eds),
'Working Class Youth Culture', Routledge & Kegan Paul.
CLARKE, R.V.G. and CORNISH, D.B. (1972) 'The Con-
trolled Trial in Institutional Research – Paradigm or Pit-
fall for Penal Evaluators', Home Office Research Studies,
15, HMSO.
CLARKE, R.V.G. and CORNISH, D.B. (1975) 'Residential
Treatment and Its Effects on Delinquency', Home Office
Research Studies, 32, HMSO.
COCKRAM, L. and BELOFF, H. (1978) 'Rehearsing to be
Adults', National Youth Bureau.
COFER, C.N. and APPLEY, M.H. (1964) 'Motivation:
Theory and Research', Wiley.
COHEN, P. (1972) Subcultural Conflict and Working Class
Community, in 'Working Papers in Cultural Studies No. 2',
University of Birmingham.
COHEN, S. (1968) The Nature of Vandalism, 'New Society',
12 December, pp. 875-8.
COHEN, S. (1972) 'Folk Devils and Moral Panics', Paladin.
COLEMAN, J.C. (1974) 'Relationships in Adolescence',
Routledge & Kegan Paul.
COLEMAN, J.C. (1978) Current Contradictions in Adoles-
cent Theory, 'Journal of Youth and Adolescence', 7.1, pp.
1-11.
COLEMAN, J.S. (1961) 'The Adolescent Society', Free
Press.
COLLINS, N. and HOGGARTH, L. (1977) 'No Man's Land-
marks', National Youth Bureau.
CONGER, J.J. (1973) 'Adolescence and Youth: Psycholo-
gical Development in a Changing World', Harper & Row.
CONGER, J.W. (1975) 'Contemporary Issues in Adolescent
Development', Harper & Row.
COOPER, D. (1971) 'The Death of the Family', Penguin.
COOPER, R. (1969) Alienation from Work, 'New Society',
30 January, pp. 161-3.
CORRIGAN, P. (1979) 'Schooling the Smash Street Kids',
Macmillan.
CORRIGAN, P. and LEONARD, P. (1978) 'Social Work
Practice Under Capitalism: a Marxist Approach', Macmillan.

COSER, R.L. (ed.) (1974) 'The Family, Its Structures and Functions', Macmillan.
COYLE, G. (1948) 'Groupwork with American Youth', American Association of Social Workers.
CRAFT, M. and CRAFT, A. (1978) 'Sex and the Mentally Handicapped', Routledge & Kegan Paul.
DANIEL, S. and MCGUIRE, P. (1972) 'The Paint House', Penguin.
DAVIES, B. (1975) The Life of Adolescence, 'New Society', 20 March, pp. 714-16.
DAVIES, K. (1974) The Sociology of Parent-Youth Conflict, in R.L. Coser (ed.), 'The Family, Its Structures and Functions', Macmillan.
DAVIES, M. (1969), 'Probationers in their Social Environment', HMSO.
DAVIES, M. (1974), 'Social Work in the Environment', HMSO.
DAVIES, M. (1977), 'Support Systems in Social Work', Routledge & Kegan Paul.
DAVIS, L.F. (1977) Feelings and Emotions in Residential Settings: the Individual Experience, 'British Journal of Social Work', 7.1, pp. 23-39.
DENNIS, N. (1958) The Popularity of the Neighbourhood Community Idea, 'Sociological Review', 6.2, pp. 191-206.
DHSS (1975), 'Hostels for Young People', Development Group Report, HMSO.
DHSS (1977a) 'Intermediate Treatment: 28 Choices', Development Group Report, HMSO.
DHSS (1977b) 'Intermediate Treatment: Planning for Action', Development Group Report, HMSO.
DHSS (1978) 'Social Services Teams: The Practitioner's View', HMSO.
DOCKER-DRYSDALE, B. (1968) 'Therapy in Child Care', Longman.
DOUGLAS, J.W.B. (1967) 'The Home and the School', Panther.
DOUGLAS, T. (1976) 'Groupwork Practice', Tavistock.
DOUVAN, E. and ADELSON, J. (1966) 'The Adolescent Experience', Wiley.
DRAKE, C.T. and MCDOUGALL, D. (1977) Effects of an Absence of a Father and Other Male Models on the Development of Boys' Sexual Roles, 'Development Psychology', 13.5, pp. 537-8.

DUHRSSEN, A. and JORSWIECK, R. (1962) Zur Korrektur von Eysenck's Berichterstattung uber Psychoanalytische Behandlung Sergebnisse, 'Acta Psychoterapeutica', 10, pp. 329-42 (a translation by Mrs K. Baker, compiled by Colin Pritchard, is available from Mr Pritchard at the University of Bath).

DUNHAM, J. (1978) Staff Stress in Residential Work, 'Social Work Today', 9.45, pp. 18-20.

DUNHAM, J., CASEY, T., SIMPSON, J. and GILLING-SMITH, D. (1976) 'Stress in Schools', NAS/UWT.

DUNLOP, A.B. (1974) 'The Approved School Experience', Home Office Research Studies, 25, HMSO.

DUNPHY, E. (1963) The Social Structure of Urban Adolescent Peer Groups, 'Sociometry', 26.2, pp. 230-46.

ECKELAAR, J., CLIVE, E., CLARKE, K. and RAIKES, S. (1977) 'Custody after Divorce', Centre for Socio-Legal Studies, Wolfson College, Oxford.

EGGLESTON, J. (1975) 'Adolescence and Community', Arnold.

EMERSON, G., MARSHALL, D. and ROBERTS, L. (1977) Rent-a-Pig, 'Youth in Society', 25, pp. 33-4.

ERIKSON, E.H. (1977) 'Childhood and Society', Paladin.

EVANS, R. (1976) Some Implications of an Integrated Model of Social Work for Theory and Practice, 'British Journal of Social Work', 6.2, pp. 177-200.

EVANS, R. (1978) Unitary Models of Practice and the Social Work Team, in M.R. Olsen (ed.), 'The Unitary Model: Its Implications for Social Work Theory and Practice', BASW.

EYSENCK, H.J. (1952) The Effects of Psychotherapy: an Evaluation, 'Journal of Consulting Psychology', 16, pp. 319-24.

EYSENCK, H.J. (1960) 'The Structure of Human Personality', Methuen.

EYSENCK, H.J. (1964) The Effects of Psychotherapy Reconsidered, 'Acta Psychotherapeutica', 12, pp. 45-52.

EYSENCK, H.J. and NIAS, D.K.B. (1978) 'Sex, Violence and the Media', Maurice Temple Smith.

EYSENCK, H.J. and RACHMAN, S. (1964) The Application of Learning Theory to Child Psychiatry, in J. Howells (ed.), 'Modern Perspectives in Child Psychiatry', Oliver & Boyd.

FARRINGTON, D.P. (1978) Family Backgrounds of Agressive Youths, in L. Hersov and M. Berger (eds), 'Aggression and Anti-Social Behaviour in Childhood and Adolescence', Pergamon.

FAUST, M.S. (1960) Developmental Maturity as a Deter-
minant in Prestige of Adolescent Girls, 'Child Develop-
ment', 31, pp. 173-84.
FERRI, E. and ROBINSON, H. (1976) 'Coping Alone',
NFER.
FERRIS, J. (1978) The Effect of Relationships with Staff
on the Attitudes and Behaviour of Delinquent Boys Under-
going Residential Intervention in an Approved School, 'The
Community Home Schools Gazette', 72.8, pp. 325-35.
FIELD, E., HAMMOND, W.H. and TIZARD, J. (1971)
'Thirteen Year Old Approved School Boys in 1962', HMSO.
FINER REPORT (1974) 'Report of the Committee on One-
Parent Families', Cmnd 5629, HMSO.
FISCHER, J. (1978) Does Anything Work?, 'Journal of
Social Service Research', 3, pp. 215-43.
FITZHERBERT, K. (1977) 'Child Care Services and the
Teacher', Maurice Temple Smith.
FOGELMAN, K. (1976a) 'Britain's Sixteen Year Olds',
National Children's Bureau.
FOGELMAN, K. (1976b) Bored Children, 'New Society',
15 July, pp. 117-18.
FORD, D. (1975) 'Children, Courts and Caring', Constable.
FOULKES, S.H. and ANTHONY, E.J. (1962) 'Group Psy-
chotherapy: the Psychoanalytic Approach', Penguin.
FOWLER, I.A. (1967) Family Agency Characteristics and
Client Continuance, 'Social Casework', 48, pp. 271-7.
FREUD, A. (1965) 'Normality and Pathology in Childhood',
Hogarth Press.
FRIEDENBURG, E. (1969) Current Patterns of Genera-
tional Conflict, 'American Journal of Sociology', 25, pp.
246-53.
FRY, A. (1978) The University of Life on a Council Estate,
'Community Care', 7 June, pp. 12-16.
GARMEZY, N. and STREITMAN, S. (1974) Children at
Risk: the Search for the Antecedents of Schizophrenia,
'Schizophrenia Bulletin', 8, pp. 14-90.
GATH, D., COOPER, B., GATTONI, F. and ROCKET, D.
(1977) 'Child Guidance and Delinquency in a London Bor-
ough', Oxford University Press.
GAY, M., COPUS, H. and HOLDER, M. (1973) Maladjust-
ment in a Large Comprehensive School, 'Bristol Education
Committee Report'.
GILL, O. (1974) Housing Policy and Neighbourhood Decline,
'Social Work Today', 5.18, pp. 558-61.
GILL, O. (1974) 'Whitegate: An Approved School in Tran-
sition', Liverpool University Press.

GILL, O. (1976) Urban Stereotypes and Delinquent Incidents, 'British Journal of Criminology', 16.4, pp. 321-36.
GILL, O. (1977) 'Luke Street', Macmillan.
GLADSTONE, F. (1979) Crime and the Crystal Ball, 'Research Bulletin No. 7', Home Office Research Unit.
GLICK, I.D. and KESSLER, D.R. (1974) 'Marital and Family Therapy', Grune & Stratton.
GOETSCHIUS, G. and TASH, J. (1967) 'Working with Unattached Youth', Routledge & Kegan Paul.
GOLAN, N. (1978) 'Treatment in Crisis Situation', Free Press.
GOLDBERG, E. and NEILL, J.E. (1972) 'Social Work in General Practice', Allen & Unwin.
GOLDSTEIN, H. (1973) 'Social Work Practice: a Unitary Approach', University of South Carolina Press.
GOLDSTEIN, J., FREUD, A. and SOLNIT, A. (1977) 'Beyond the Best Interests of the Child', Free Press.
GREGORY, W.H. (1980) Secure Provision for Children and Young People, in R.G. Walton and D. Elliot (eds), 'Residential Care: A Reader in Current Theory and Practice', Pergamon.
GRUNSELL, R. (1976) Educational Aspects of Intermediate Treatment, in DHSS Development Group (eds), 'Intermediate Treatment', HMSO.
GULBENKIAN FOUNDATION STUDY GROUP ON TRAINING (1968) 'Community Work and Social Change', Longman.
HALL, A. (1974) 'The Point of Entry: A Study of Client Perceptions in the Social Services', Allen & Unwin.
HALL, A. (1975) Policy-Making: More Judgement than Luck, 'Community Care', 6 August, pp. 16-18.
HALLECK, S. (1963) The Impact of Professional Dishonesty on the Behaviour of Disturbed Adolescents, 'Social Work', 8.2, pp. 48-56.
HALMOS, P. (1978) 'The Personal and the Political', Hutchinson.
HARE, R.D. and SCHALLING, D. (eds) (1978) 'Psychopathic Behaviour: Approaches to Research', Wiley.
HARGREAVES, D.H. (1967) 'Social Relations in a Secondary School', Routledge & Kegan Paul.
HARGREAVES, D.H., HESTOR, S.K. and MELLOR, F.J. (1975) 'Deviance in Classrooms', Routledge & Kegan Paul.
HARLOW, H. (1958) The Nature of Love, 'American Psychologist', 13, p. 673.
HEAP, K. (1977) 'Group Theory for Social Workers', Pergamon.

HEAP, K. (1979) 'Process and Action in Work with Groups', Pergamon.
HEARN, G. (ed.) (1969) 'The General Systems Approach: Contributions Toward an Holistic Conception of Social Work', Council on Social Work Education.
HERBERT, W.L. and JARVIS, F.V. (1961) 'Dealing with Delinquents', Methuen.
HERON, J. (1975) 'Six Category Intervention Analysis', University of Surrey.
HERSOV, L. (1960) Persistent Non-Attendance at School: Refusal to Go to School, 'Journal of Child Psychology and Psychiatry', 1, pp. 130-6.
HERZBERG, F. (1968) 'Work and the Nature of Man', Wiley.
HINDLELANG, M.J. (1976) With a Little Help from Their Friends: Participation in Reported Delinquent Behaviour, 'British Journal of Criminology', 16.2, pp. 109-25.
HODGE, J. (1977) Social Groupwork - Rules for Establishing the Group, 'Social Work Today', 18.17, pp. 8-10.
HOGHUGHI, M.S. (1978a) Democracy and Delinquency, 'British Journal of Criminology', 18.4, pp. 391-6.
HOGHUGHI, M.S. (1978b) 'Troubled and Troublesome: Coping with Severely Disturbed Children', André Deutsch.
HOLLIS, F. (1974) 'Casework - a Psychosocial Therapy', Random House.
HOLMAN, R. (1975) The Place of Fostering in Social Work, 'British Journal of Social Work', 5.1, pp. 3-29.
HOME OFFICE (1970) 'Part I of the Children and Young Persons Act 1969 - a Guide for Courts and Practitioners', HMSO.
HOUSE OF COMMONS EXPENDITURE COMMITTEE (1975) 'Eleventh Report: the Children and Young Persons Act, vols 1 and 2, HMSO.
HUDSON, J. (1978) In Residence, 'Social Work Today', 9.20, p. 23.
HUDSON, J. (1979) The Heart of Social Work, 'Social Work Today', 10.41, p. 17.
HUMPHRIES, K. (1977) Number 5 - a counselling service for young people, 'Youth in Society', 22, p. 24.
HUNTER, J. and AINSWORTH, F. (eds) (1975) 'A Unitary Approach to Social Work Practice - Implications for Education and Organisation', School of Social Administration, University of Dundee.
HUTTEN, J.M. (1977) 'Short-Term Contracts in Social Work', Routledge & Kegan Paul.

INHELDER, B. and PIAGET, J. (1958) 'The Growth of
Logical Thinking', Routledge & Kegan Paul.
JACKSON, B. and MARSDEN, D. (1966) 'Education and
the Working Class', Penguin.
JAHODA, M. (1979) The Psychological Meanings of Unem-
ployment, 'New Society', 19 January, pp. 492-5.
JANCHILL, SISTER M.P. (1969) Systems Concepts in Case-
work Theory and Practice, 'Social Casework', 50, pp. 74-82.
JEHU, D., HARDIKER, P., YELLOLY, I.M. and SHAW, M.
(1972) 'Behaviour Modification in Social Work', Wiley.
JONES, A. (1976) The Single Parent Child in the Inner City
School, 'Concern', 20, pp. 12-19.
JONES, C.O. (1977) Disruption and Disturbance: observa-
tions on the management of a group of junior school-age
children, 'Concern', 25, pp. 7-21.
JONES, H. (1979) 'The Residential Community', Routledge
& Kegan Paul.
JONES, R. (1976) Getting IT Together: integrating inter-
mediate treatment, 'Social Work Today', 7.5, pp. 130-5.
JONES, R. (1979) 'Fun and Therapy: Consumer and Social
Worker Perceptions of Intermediate Treatment', National
Youth Bureau.
JONES, R. and KERSLAKE, A. (1979) 'Intermediate Treat-
ment and Social Work', Heinemann.
JONES, R. and WALTER, T. (1978) Delinquency is Fun,
'Community Care', 9 August, pp. 20-1.
JORDAN, W. (1972) 'The Social Worker in Family Situa-
tions', Routledge & Kegan Paul.
JOSSELYN, I. (1952) 'The Adolescent and His World',
Family Service Association of America.
KAHAN, B. (ed.) (1977) 'Working Together for Children and
their Families', HMSO.
KAHN, J. and NURSTEN, J. (1964) 'Unwillingly to
School', Pergamon.
KENNY, B. and WHITEHEAD, T. (1973) 'Insight', Croom
Helm.
KING, L.G. (1972) Affective Syndromes in Normal Young
People, 'Diseases of the Nervous System', 33, pp. 736-41.
KLINE, P. (1972) 'Fact and Fantasy in Freudian Theory',
Methuen.
KNIGHT, L. (1977) One Alternative to Residential Care,
'Community Care', 20 July, pp. 16-17.
KOGAN, L.S. (1957) 'Study of Short-term Cases at a
Community Service Centre', Institute of Welfare Research,
New York.

KONOPKA, G. (1963) 'Social Group Work', Prentice-Hall.
KREITMAN, N. (ed.) (1977) 'Parasuicide', Wiley.
LAING, R.D. (1960) 'The Divided Self', Penguin.
LAING, R.D. and ESTERSON, A. (1964) 'Sanity, Madness and the Family', Penguin.
LAMBERT, L. and HART, S. (9176) Who Needs a Father?, 'New Society', 8 July, p. 80.
LANDSBAUM, J.B. and WILLIS, R.H. (1971) Conformity in Early and Late Adolescence, 'Developmental Psychology', 4.3, pp. 334-7.
LANG, T. (1974) Alienated Children: Psychologies of School Phobia and their Social and Political Indication, in N. Armistead (ed.), 'Restructuring Social Psychology', Penguin.
LARSON, L.E. (1975) The Relative Influence of Parent-Adolescent Affect, in J.J. Conger (ed.), 'Contemporary Issues in Adolescent Development', Harper & Row.
LAUFER, M. (1975) 'Adolescent Disturbance and Breakdown', Penguin.
LAZARUS, A.A. (1976) 'Multi-Modal Behaviour Therapy', Springer.
LEFRANÇOIS, G.R. (1976) 'Adolescents', Wadsworth.
LEISSNER, A., POWLEY, T. and EVANS, D. (1977) 'Intermediate Treatment', National Children's Bureau.
LERMAN, P. (1975) 'Community Treatment and Social Control', University of Chicago Press.
LESSER, G. and KANDEL, D. (1969) Parent-Adolescent Relationships, 'Journal of Marriage and the Family', 31, pp. 62-74.
LICCIONE, J.V. (1955) The Changing Family Relationships of Adolescent Girls, 'Journal of Abnormal and Social Psychology', 51, pp. 421-6.
LIPPITT, R., WATSON, J. and WESTLEY, B. (1958) 'The Dynamics of Planned Change', Harcourt, Brace & World.
LIPTON, D., MARTINSON, R. and WILKS, J. (1975) 'The Effectiveness of Correctional Treatment', Praeger.
LOVELL, K. (1973) 'Introduction to Human Development', Macmillan.
MACK, J. (1976) Children Half Alone, 'New Society', 7 October, pp. 19-23.
MACK, J. (1977) West Indians and School, 'New Society', 8 December, pp. 510-12.
MACKLENNAN, B.W. and FELSENDFELDT, N. (1968) 'Group Counselling and Psychotherapy with Adolescents', Columbia University Press.

MADDOX, B. (1975) 'The Half-Parent: Living with Other People's Children', André Deutsch.
MARCHANT, H. and SMITH, M. (1977) 'Adolescent Girls at Risk', Pergamon.
MARSDEN, D. (1973) 'Mothers Alone', Penguin.
MARSH, P. (1978) Football Hooliganism, 'Inter-action Press'.
MARSHALL, T. (1976) Vandalism: the Seeds of Destruction, 'New Society', 17 June, pp. 625-7.
MARTINSON, R. (1974) What Works? - Questions and Answers About Prison Reform, 'Public Interest', Spring, pp. 22-52.
MASLOW, A.H. (1968) 'Towards a Psychology of Being', Van Nostrand.
MASLOW, A.H. (1970) 'Motivation and Personality', Harper & Row.
MASTERSON, J.F. (1967) 'The Psychiatric Dilemma of Adolescence', Little Brown.
MATHIESON, D. (1975) Conflict and Change in Probation, 'Probation Journal', 22.2, pp. 36-41.
MATZA, D. (1964) 'Delinquency and Drift', Wiley.
MAYER, J.E. and TIMMS, N. (1970) 'The Client Speaks', Routledge & Kegan Paul.
MAYS, J.B. (1954) 'Growing Up in the City', Liverpool University Press.
MAYS, J.B. (1965) 'The Young Pretenders', Sphere.
MAYS, J.B. (1972) Delinquency and the Transition from School to Work, in J.B. Mays (ed.), 'Juvenile Delinquency, the Family and the Social Group', Longman.
MCCULLOCH, W. and PHILIP, A.E. (1972) 'Suicidal Behaviour', Pergamon.
MCGREGOR, D. (1960) 'The Human Side of Enterprise', McGraw-Hill.
MEEKS, J. (1971) 'The Fragile Alliance', Williams & Wilkins.
MENNINGER, K. (1963) 'The Vital Balance', Viking Press.
MERRISON REPORT (1979) 'Report of the Royal Commission on the NHS', Cmnd 7615, HMSO.
MEYER, H. (1976) 'Social Work Practice: The Changing Landscape', Free Press.
MIDDLEMAN, R.R. and GOLDBERG, G. (1973) 'Social Service Delivery: A Structural Approach to Social Work Practice', Columbia University Press.
MILLER, W. (1958) Lower Class Life as a Generating Milieu of Gang Delinquency, 'Journal of Social Issues', 14.3, pp. 5-19.

MILLHAM, S., BULLOCK, R. and CHERRETT, P. (1975) 'After Grace – Teeth', Chaucer.

MILLHAM, S., BULLOCK, R. and HOSIE, K. (1978) 'Locking-up Children', Saxon House.

MITTLER, P. (1971) 'The Study of Twins', Penguin.

MORSE, M. (1965) 'The Unattached', Penguin.

MUSGROVE, F. (1964) 'Youth and the Social Order', Routledge & Kegan Paul.

MUSSEN, P.H., CONGER, J.J. and KAGAN, J. (1974) 'Child Development and Personality', Harper & Row.

NEWMAN, O. (1972) 'Defensible Space', Architectural Press.

NEWSOM, J. and NEWSOM, E. (1963) 'Infant Care in an Urban Community', Allen & Unwin.

NEWSOM, J. and NEWSOM, E. (1968) 'Four Years Old in an Urban Community', Allen & Unwin.

NICHOLS, W. and RUTLEDGE, A. (1965) Psychotherapy with Teenagers, 'Journal of Marriage and the Family', 27.2, pp. 166–76.

NORMAN, J. (1977) 870 House IT Unit, in DHSS (eds), 'Intermediate Treatment: 28 Choices', HMSO.

NORTHERN, H. (1969) 'Social Work with Groups', Columbia University Press.

NURSTEN, J.P. (1974) 'The Process of Casework', Pitman.

NUTTALL, E.V., NUTTALL, R.L., POLIT, D. and CLARK, K. (1977) Assessing Adolescents' Mental Health Needs: The Views of Consumers, Providers and Others, 'Adolescence', 12.46, pp. 277–85.

OFFER, D., MARCUS, D. and OFFER, J. (1970) A Longitudinal Study of Normal Adolescent Boys, 'American Journal of Psychiatry', 126, pp. 917–24.

OFFER, D. and OFFER, J. (1969) 'The Psychological World of the Teenager', Basic Books.

OFFER, D. and OFFER, J.L. (1969) Grown-up: A Follow-up Study of Normal Adolescents, 'Seminar Psychiatric', 1.1, pp. 46–56.

OPCS (1969), quoted in B. Hudson (1978) Overhauling the Youth Service, 'Community Care', 2 August, pp. 18–19.

PACKMAN, J. (1975) 'The Child's Generation', Blackwell & Robertson.

PAGAN, A. (1978) A Capital Venture: Promoting Intermediate Treatment in London, 'Social Work Service', 16, DHSS.

PAGE, R. and CLARK, G.A. (eds) (1977) 'Who Cares? Young People in Care Speak Out', National Children's Bureau.

PARKER, H. (1974) 'View from the Boys', David & Charles.
PARKER, R.A. (1971) 'Planning for Deprived Children', National Children's Home.
PAYNE, C. (1977) Improving Teamwork, 'Social Work Today', 9.1, p. 26.
PAYNE, C. (1978) Groups in the Residential Setting, in N. McCaughan (ed.), 'Groupwork: Learning and Practice', Routledge & Kegan Paul.
PAYNE, L. (1976) Interdisciplinary Experiment, 'Social Work Today', 6.22, pp. 691-3.
PEARSON, G. (1978) Leisure, Popular Culture and Street Games, 'Youth in Society', 30, pp. 4-7.
PERSONAL SOCIAL SERVICES COUNCIL (1977) 'A Future for Intermediate Treatment', PSSC.
PHILIPS, M. (1976) Brixton and Crime, 'New Society', 8 July, pp. 65-8.
PINCKERTON, P. (1974) 'Psychosomatic Approach to Childhood Disorder', Crosby Lockwood Staples.
PINCUS, A. and MINAHAN, A. (1973) 'Social Work Practice: Model and Method', Peacock.
PINCUS, A. and MINAHAN, A. (1977) A Model for Social Work Practice, in H. Specht and A. Vickery (eds) 'Integrating Social Work Methods', Allen & Unwin.
PLANT, R. (1974) 'Community and Ideology', Routledge & Kegan Paul.
POWER, M.J., ALDERSON, M.R., PHILLIPSON, C.M., SHOENBERG, E. and MORRIS, J.N. (1967) Delinquent Schools?, 'New Society', 19 October, pp. 542-3.
PRINGLE, M.L.K. (1967) '11,000 Seven Year Olds', Longmans.
PRINGLE, M.L.K. (1974) 'The Needs of Children', Hutchinson.
PRINS, H.A. (1973) 'Criminal Behaviour', Pitman Press.
PRITCHARD, C. (1974) The Education Welfare Officer, Truancy and School Phobia, 'Social Work Today', 5.5, pp. 130-4.
PRITCHARD, C. and BUTLER, A. (1978) Teachers' Perceptions of School Phobic and Truant Behaviour and the Influence of the Youth Tutor, 'Journal of Adolescence', 1.4, pp. 273-82.
PRITCHARD, C. and TAYLOR, R.K.S. (1978) Perceptions of Violence in Schools, 'Therapeutic Education', 6.2, pp. 4-11.
PRITCHARD, C. and TAYLOR, R.K.S. (1978) 'Social Work: Reform or Revolution?', Routledge & Kegan Paul.

Young People in Care Speak Out', National Children's
Bureau.
PARKER, H. (1974) 'View from the Boys', David & Charles.
PARKER, R.A. (1971) 'Planning for Deprived Children',
National Children's Home.
PAYNE, C. (1977) Improving Teamwork, 'Social Work
Today', 9.1, p. 26.
PAYNE, C. (1978) Groups in the Residential Setting, in
N. McCaughan (ed.), 'Groupwork: Learning and Practice',
Routledge & Kegan Paul.PAYNE, L. (1976) Interdisciplin-
ary Experiment, 'Social Work Today', 6.22, pp. 691-3.
PEARSON, G. (1978) Leisure, Popular Culture and Street
Games, 'Youth in Society', 30, pp. 4-7.
PERSONAL SOCIAL SERVICES COUNCIL (1977) 'A Future
for Intermediate Treatment', PSSC.
PHILIPS, M. (1976) Brixton and Crime, 'New Society',
8 July, pp. 65-8.
PINCKERTON, P. (1974) 'Psychosomatic Approach to
Childhood Disorder', Crosby Lockwood Staples.
PINCUS, A. and MINAHAN, A. (1973) 'Social Work Prac-
tice: Model and Method', Peacock.
PINCUS, A. and MINAHAN, A. (1977) A Model for Social
Work Practice, in H. Specht and A. Vickery (eds), 'Inte-
grating Social Work Methods', Allen & Unwin.
PLANT, R. (1974) 'Community and Ideology', Routledge &
Kegan Paul.
POWER, M.J., ALDERSON, M.R., PHILLIPSON, C.M.,
SHOENBERG, E. and MORRIS, J.N. (1967) Delinquent
Schools?, 'New Society', 19 October, pp. 542-3.
PRINGLE, M.L.K. (1967) '11,000 Seven Year Olds',
Longmans.
PRINGLE, M.L.K. (1974) 'The Needs of Children',
Hutchinson.
PRINS, H.A. (1973) 'Criminal Behaviour', Pitman Press.
PRITCHARD, C. (1974) The Education Welfare Officer,
Truancy and School Phobia, 'Social Work Today', 5.5,
pp. 130-4.
PRITCHARD, C. and BUTLER, A. (1978) Teachers' Per-
ceptions of School Phobic and Truant Behaviour and the
Influence of the Youth Tutor, 'Journal of Adolescence',
1.4, pp. 273-82.
PRITCHARD, C. and TAYLOR, R.K.S. (1978) Perceptions
of Violence in Schools, 'Therapeutic Education', 6.2,
pp. 4-11.
PRITCHARD, C. and TAYLOR, R.K.S. (1978) 'Social
Work - Reform or Revolution?', Routledge & Kegan Paul.

240 Bibliography

PRITCHARD, C. and TAYLOR, R.K.S. (1979) Inter-professional Perceptions of Violence in Schools: a comparison
of teachers' and social workers' views, 'Occasional Paper
No. I', Centre for Social Work and Applied Social Studies,
University of Leeds.
PRITCHARD, C., TAYLOR, R.K.S. and KING, R.L.
(1978) Relations between Caring Professions, 'British
Association for the Advancement of Science Annual Confer-
ence', University of Bath, September.
PRITCHARD, C. and WARD, R.I. (1974) Family Dynamics
of School Phobics, 'British Journal of Social Work', 4.1,
pp. 61-94.
PRYCE, K. (1979) 'Endless Pressure', Penguin.
RADIN, S.S. (1967) Psychodynamic Aspects of School
Phobia, 'Comprehensive Psychiatry', 8.2, pp. 119-28.
RAPAPORT, L. (1970) Crisis Intervention as a Model of
Brief Treatment, in R.W. Roberts and R.H. Nee (eds),
'Theories of Social Casework', University of Chicago
Press.
RATOFF, L., ROSE, A. and SMITH, C.R. (1974) Social
Workers and GPs, 'Social Work Today', 5.16, pp. 8-10.
REDL, F. (1975) Introduction, in M. Sugar (ed.), 'The
Adolescent in Group and Family Therapy', Bruner/Mazel.
REES, S. (1978) 'Social Work Face to Face', Arnold.
REID, K. (1977) Nonrational Dynamics of the Client-Worker
Interaction, 'Social Casework', 58.10.
REID, W.J. and EPSTEIN, L. (1972) 'Task-Centred Case-
work', Columbia University Press.
REID, W.J. and EPSTEIN, L. (1977) 'Task-Centred Prac-
tice', Columbia University Press.
REID, W.J. and SHYNE, A. (1969) 'Brief and Extended
Casework', Columbia University Press.
REYNOLDS, D. (1976) When Pupils and Teachers Refuse a
Truce: the Secondary School and the Creation of Delin-
quency, in G. Mungham and G. Pearson (eds), 'Working
Class Youth Culture', Routledge & Kegan Paul.
REYNOLDS, D. and JONES, D. (1978) Education and the
Prevention of Juvenile Delinquency, in N. Tutt (ed.), 'Al-
ternative Strategies for Coping with Crime', Blackwell &
Robertson.
ROBINS, D. and COHEN, P. (1978) 'Knuckle Sandwich',
Penguin.
ROBINSON, M. (1978) 'Schools and Social Work', Rout-
ledge & Kegan Paul.
ROBINSON, T. (1978) 'In Worlds Apart', Bedford Square
Press.

ROGERS, C.R. (1962) 'On Becoming A Person', Houghton Mifflin.
ROGERS, C.R. (1971) The Process Equation in Psychotherapy, in J.T. Hart and T.M. Tomlinson (eds), 'New Directions in Client-Centred Therapy', Houghton Mifflin.
ROSE, G. and MARSHALL, T.F. (1974) 'Counselling and School Social Work', Wiley.
ROWNTREE, M. (1965) An Introduction to Intermediate Treatment, 'Probation', 17.1, pp. 18-21.
RUTHERFORD, A. (1977) 'Youth Crime Policy in the United States', Institute for the Study and Treatment of Delinquency.
RUTTER, M. (1971) Normal Psychosexual Development, 'Journal of Child Psychology and Psychiatry', II, pp. 259-83.
RUTTER, M. (1974) A Child's Life, 'New Scientist', 27 June.
RUTTER, M. (1975) 'Helping Troubled Children', Penguin.
RUTTER, M. (1977) Protective Factors in Children in Response to Stress and Disadvantage, '3rd Vermont Conference', University of Vermont, June.
RUTTER, M. (1978) Research into Prevention of Psychosocial Disorders in Childhood, in J. Barnes and N. Connelly (eds), 'Social Care Research', Bedford Square Press.
RUTTER, M. and GRAHAM, P. (1968) The Reliability and Validity of the Psychiatric Assessment of the Child, 'British Journal of Psychiatry', 114, pp. 563-79.
RUTTER, M., GRAHAM, P., CHADWICK, O. and YULE, W. (1976) Adolescent Turmoil: Fact or Fiction?, 'Journal of Child Psychology and Psychiatry', 17, pp. 35-56.
RUTTER, M., MAUGHAN, B., MORTIMORE, P., and OUSTON, J. (1979) 'Fifteen Thousand Hours', Open Books.
SAINSBURY, E. (1975) 'Social Work with Families', Routledge & Kegan Paul.
SANDSTROM, C.I. (1966) 'The Psychology of Childhood and Adolescence', Methuen.
SATIR, V. (1967) 'Conjoint Family Therapy', Science and Behaviour Books.
SCHONFELD, W. (1967) Adolescent Psychiatry, 'Archives of General Psychiatry', 16.6, pp. 713-19.
SEGAL, S.P. (1972) Research on the Outcome of Social Work Therapeutic Interventions: a Review of the Literature, 'Journal of Health and Social Behaviour', 13.1, pp. 3-17.
SELIGMAN, M.E.P. (1975) 'Learned Helplessness', Freeman.

SHAPLAND, J.M. (1978) Self Reported Delinquency in Boys aged 11 to 14, 'British Journal of Criminology', 18.3, pp. 255-66.

SHEEHY, G. (1977) 'Passages: Predictable Crisis of Adult Life', Bantam.

SHEPHERD, G. and RICHARDSON, A. (1979) Social Skills Training and Beyond, 'Behavioural Psychotherapy', 7.2, pp. 31-8.

SHERIF, M. (1967) 'Group Conflict and Co-operation', Routledge & Kegan Paul.

SKYNNER, A.C.R. (1974) An Experiment in Group Consultation with the Staff of a Comprehensive School, 'Group Process', 66, pp. 99-114.

SMALE, G. (1977) 'Prophecy, Behaviour and Change', Routledge & Kegan Paul.

SMITH, C.S., FARRANT, M.R. and MARCHANT, H.J. (1972) 'The Wincroft Youth Project', Tavistock.

SMITH, R.M. and WATTERS, J. (1978) Delinquent and Non-delinquent Males' Perceptions of their Fathers, 'Adolescence', 13.49, pp. 21-8.

SMITH, T.E. (1974) Push Versus Pull: intra-family versus peer-group variables as possible determinants of adolescent orientations toward parents, 'Youth and Society', 8.1, pp. 5-26.

'SOCIAL TRENDS' (1979) HMSO.

SPECHT, H. and VICKERY, A. (eds) (1977) 'Integrating Social Work Methods', Allen & Unwin.

SPENCER, J. (1964) 'Stress and Release in an Urban Estate', Tavistock.

SPINETTA, J.J. and RIGLER, D. (1972) The Child Abusing Parent: A Psychological Review, 'Psychological Bulletin', 77.4, pp. 296-304.

STIERLIN, H. (1975) Countertransference in Family Therapy with Adolescence, in M. Sugar (ed.), 'The Adolescent in Group and Family Therapy', Bruner/Mazel.

STOTT, D.H. (1966) 'Manual to the Bristol Social Adjustment Guides', 3rd edition, University of London Press.

STRATTA, E. (1970) 'The Education of Borstal Boys', Routledge & Kegan Paul.

TANNER, J.M. (1962) 'Growth at Adolescence', Blacwell.

TANNER, J.M. (1970) Physical Growth, in P.H. Mussey (ed.), 'Carmichael's Manual of Child Psychology', Wiley.

TAYLOR, I. (1971) Soccer Consciousness and Soccer Hooliganism, in S. Cohen (ed.), 'Images of Deviance', Penguin.

TAYLOR, I. and WALL, D. (1976) Beyond the Skinheads: Comments on the Emergence and Significance of the Glamrock Cult, in G. Mungham and G. Pearson (eds), 'Working Class Youth Culture', Routledge & Kegan Paul.

TENNAL SCHOOL (1976) Assessment, Management and Evaluation Manual, Tennal School, Birmingham, unpublished.

THOMAS, A., CHESS, S. and BIRCH, R.G. (1970) The Origins of Personality, 'Scientific American', 223.2, pp. 102-9.

THOMAS, A. and CHESS, S. (1977) 'Temperament and Development', Raven Press.

THORPE, D. (1972) Putting Theory into Practice at Ryehill, 'Social Work Today', 3.1, pp. 23-5.

THORPE, D. (1977) Face to Face with Adolescents, 'Social Work Today', 8.26, pp. 16-19.

THORPE, D., PALEY, J. and GREEN, C. (1979) The Making of a Delinquent, 'Community Care', 26 April, pp. 18-19.

THORPE, D., PALEY, J. and GREEN, C. (1979) Ensuring the Right Result, 'Community Care', 10 May, pp. 25-6.

TIMMS, N. (1972) 'Recording in Social Work', Routledge & Kegan Paul.

TIMMS, N. (1975) General editorial, in H. Jones (ed.), 'Towards a New Social Work', Routledge & Kegan Paul.

TIMMS, N. and TIMMS, R. (1977) 'Perspectives in Social Work', Routledge & Kegan Paul.

TOMKINS, G. (1978) Under 21 - Young Person's Counselling and Information Centre, 'Youth in Society', 27, pp. 23-5.

TRUAX, B. and CARKUFF, C. (1967) 'Towards Effective Counselling and Psychotherapy: Training and Practice', Aldine.

TRUCKLE, B. and SCHARDT, E. (1975) Notes on Counselling Group for Adolescents, 'Group Analysis', 8.3, pp. 21-4.

TURNER, B. (1974) 'Truancy', Ward Lock.

TUTT, N. (1974) 'Care or Custody', Darton, Longman & Todd.

UTTING, W. (1977) Dealing with Delinquents in Open and Closed Conditions, 'Community Home Schools Gazette', 72.9, pp. 372-9.

VINTER, R.D. (1967) Program Activities: an analysis of their effects on participant behaviour, in P.H. Glasser, R.C. Sarris and R.D. Vinter (eds), 'Individual Change Through Small Groups', Free Press.

244 Bibliography

WALROND-SKINNER, S. (1976) 'Family Therapy – The
Treatment of Natural Systems' Routledge & Kegan Paul.
WALTER, A.J. (1978) 'Sent Away: A Study of Young
Offenders in Care', Saxon House.
WARD, D. (1977) Broadening IT Practice – the 'Child-in-
his-Living Situation', 'Social Work Today', 8.19, pp. 10-
11.
WATERHOUSE, J. (1978) Groupwork in Intermediate
Treatment, 'British Journal of Social Work', 8.2, pp. 127-
44.
WEST, D.J. (1967) 'The Young Offender', Penguin.
WEST, D.J. and FARRINGTON, D.P. (1973) 'Who Becomes
Delinquent?', Heinemann.
WEST, D.J. and FARRINGTON, D.P. (1977) 'The Delin-
quent Way of Life', Heinemann.
WHITE, R. and BROCKINGTON, D. (1978) 'In and Out of
School – the ROSLA Community Education Project',
Routledge & Kegan Paul.
WHITLAM, M.R. (1977) The Hammersmith Project, 'Social
Work Today', 9.18, pp. 7-9.
WILKINSON, R. (1966) Sleeps and Dreams, in B.M. Foss
(ed.), 'New Horizons in Psychology', Penguin.
WILLIS, P. (1977) 'Learning to Labour', Saxon House.
WILLS, D. (1971) 'Spare the Child', Penguin.
WILLMOTT, P. (1966) 'Adolescent Boys of East London',
Penguin.
WILLSON, M. (1978) The Pragmatics of Groupwork in
Social Work, 'Social Work Today', 10.14, pp. 12-15.
WILLSON, H. (1974) Parenting in Poverty, 'British Jour-
nal of Social Work', 4.3, pp. 241-54.
WILSON, H. and HERBERT, G.W. (1974) Social Depriva-
tion and Performance at School, 'Policy and Politics',
3.2, pp. 55-69.
WILSON, H. and HERBERT, G.W. (1978) 'Parents
and Children in the Inner City', Routledge & Kegan
Paul.
WINNICOTT, C. (1964) 'Child Care and Social Work',
Codicote Press.
WINNICOTT, D.W. (1960) The Theory of the Parent-
Infant Relationship, in D.W. Winnicott (ed.), 'The Matura-
tional Process and the Facilitating Environment', Hogarth
Press, 1972.
WOODROOFE, K. (1962) 'From Charity to Social Work',
Routledge & Kegan Paul.
WOOLF, S. (1967), 'Children Under Stress', Penguin.

WORKING PARTY ON MARRIAGE GUIDANCE (1979)
'Marriage Matters', HMSO.

Index

adolescence: development, 1, 5, 51, biological, 12, 21-2, emotional, 13, 20, 21, 51, 109, intellectual, 20, 25-7, 48, 110, sexual, 12, 15, 20, 22, 24-5, 48, 110-11, 116, 217-18, social, 21, 109; disturbance during, 1, 15, 91, 108, 209-10; models of, 11-19, 47-8, constitutional, 12-14, identity crisis, 14-15, 27, needs hierarchy, 16-17, social learning, 15-16, stress, 19-22, 49
adolescent(s): concerns of, 23, 25, 29, 34-6, 110, 217-18; identity, 14-15, 18, 38, 109-10, 129, 141, 166; physique, 12, 22-4, 218; rebellion, 28, 217; sexuality, 113, 116, 215; status, economic, 44-5, 109, 110, legal, 21, 46-7, 49, peer group, 24-5, 38, 113, 166, 204, social, 115-16; stress, 1, 19-22, 27, 29, 45, 107, 115-20, 210; temperament, 12, 13-14
advocacy, 53, 56, 57, 59, 60, 135
aggression, 15-16, 17, 18,

19, 48, 117, 203
assessment, 2, 20, 50, 52, 53, 58-60, 66, 67, 72, 81, 88, 107, 114, 126, 209-10; residential, 194-6
attitudes, adult-adolescent, 27, 174, 182, 183, 184

behaviour modification, 128, 196, 221

casework, 53-5, 56, 57, 58, 62, 63, 64, 145, 157, 176
child guidance service, 54, 95-6, 99, 123-4, 145
Children and Young Persons Act (1969), 59, 80, 187, 189, 190
communication, inter-professional, 85-103, 120, 164
community, concept of, 172; see also neighbourhood
community homes, 162-3; definition of, 180-1, 186-7; expectations of, 187-8
community service, 182-3
community work, 53, 54, 56-7, 58, 63, 64, 68, 76, 83, 84, 172, 176

Printed in the United States
by Baker & Taylor Publisher Services

Printed in the United States
by Baker & Taylor Publisher Services